Flat-Belly **365**

The Gut-Friendly Superfood Plan to
Shed Pounds, Fight Inflammation,
and Feel Great All Year Long

Manuel Villacorta, MS, RD

Health Communications, Inc.
Deerfield Beach, Florida

www.hcibooks.com

Library of Congress Cataloging-in-Publication Data
is available through the Library of Congress

ISBN-13: 978-07573-2010-1 (Paperback)
ISBN-10: 07573-2010-4 (Paperback)
ISBN-13: 978-07573-2011-8 (ePub)
ISBN-10: 07573-2011-2 (ePub)

Publisher: Health Communications, Inc.
        3201 S.W. 15th Street
        Deerfield Beach, FL 33442–8190

Cover photo © Manuel Villacorta
Cover design by Larissa Hise Henoch
Interior design and formatting by Lawna Patterson Oldfield

Cook

_3,00_

CONTENTS

Acknowledgments..v

Introduction 1

CHAPTER 1 The Secret to Success:
Gut-Friendly Superfoods.....................................5

CHAPTER 2 The Flat-Belly 365 Plan...................................... 15

CHAPTER 3 The 7-Day Spring Reboot..................................41

CHAPTER 4 The 7-Day Summer Reboot 63

CHAPTER 5 The 7-Day Fall Reboot 87

CHAPTER 6 The 7-Day Winter Reboot 107

CHAPTER 7 Staples, Sides, and Desserts
for All Seasons.. 129

CHAPTER 8 Beyond Flat-Belly 365—
Long-Term Success and Maintenance............. 147

About the Author 181

Index 183

ACKNOWLEDGMENTS

I wish to thank the following people, without whom I could not have completed this project. Allison Janse, my editor at HCI Books, for continuing to believe in the project. Given that this is my fourth book with her, she continues to believe in me and inspire me throughout this process. Kim Weiss, a publicist extraordinaire, who goes above and beyond. Thank you to Ian Briggs and Shyanne Solivan for your dedication, creativity, and enthusiasm in testing my recipes and helping with social media.

I would also like to thank my office team whose dedication and support allowed me to focus on the project: Uriel Serrano, who spent many hours in the kitchen creating recipes and food styling. Also supporting me with the written content of this book: Alejandro Pinot for his amazing support and creative eye and food photography, and for making sure the lighting was perfect so that pictures always looked mouthwatering. I am grateful to Destini Moody for her outstanding energy and effort with recipe nutrient analysis and assistance with meal plan development. Without all of their work, I could not have done mine. I am always grateful to my partner Jeff, the best guinea pig, and my family for their continuous support and believing in my dreams.

INTRODUCTION

As a dietitian with 18 years of experience and an author of 3 nutrition and wellness books, I have helped thousands of people reach their weight loss goals. I have done so by teaching and creating programs that use the latest findings in the field of nutrition and turning them into practical and innovative meal plans. In the last few years, I developed a program that includes my latest research in nutrition and gut health. Within this program, you will learn to incorporate several different foods, such as anti-inflammatory fats to help reduce visceral fat and superfoods for antioxidant and antiaging powers. The program also includes prebiotic and probiotic foods to keep your gut happy and healthy. This plan focuses more on the quality of food rather than counting calories.

In my private practice in San Francisco, I have been using these meal plans with my clients, and the results are outstanding. All of the clients have successfully lost weight and inches around their waists, with an average weight loss of 4 to 6 pounds within the 7-day Flat-Belly reboot week. The more they followed the plan in detail, the better the results. In addition to the weight loss, the overall health effects have been nothing short of amazing. Nearly all my clients have reported that they feel more energized, are enjoying better sleep, and feel less bloated. Here are some success stories:

Stephanie, a 50-year-old who, for the life of her, couldn't shake even a pound and kept blaming premenopause, said, *"I finally lost weight by sticking to the 1,300 calorie Spring Plan. That's truly progress! 3 pounds in one week and I don't feel bloated!"*

Sofia, a 62-year-old, couldn't lose any weight, even by cutting out carbs. She lost 15 pounds and 3 inches around her waist by using 2 weeks of the Winter Plan and two weeks of the Spring Plan back to back. *"This morning I was able to put on two skirts and close the clasp on the waist!"*

Jeff, a 35-year-old, tried all four of the seasonal meal plans within 3 months and posted on Facebook, *"Woo hoo! Almost 23 pounds dropped! It was so easy and delicious. Thanks for the tools."*

The simple science behind weight loss is that you *do* need to cut calories; however, now that we know more about nutrition and gut health, we know that it doesn't stop there. For the calories you do consume, it really does matter which foods they come from, because the food you eat can really have an effect on your health and, most importantly, your gut. Certain foods can potentially upset the balance of microbes in your gut, as well as contribute to the formation of visceral fat or abdominal fat. Visceral fat is the type of fat that surrounds your organs and is the worst fat to carry around your waistline, since it is the cause of inflammation, the source of many other chronic diseases. I will discuss chronic inflammation, the types of body fat, and their effects on the human body in Chapter 1.

Even if you are losing weight but are not eating the right foods, your diet alone can create inflammation, regardless of the level of visceral fat or the balance of your gut bacteria. This is where superfoods can help, because they are anti-inflammatory foods that are packed with antioxidants that help reduce inflammation.

In this book, I have developed meal plans that take away the thinking and make it easier to incorporate these foods into your life. With *Flat-Belly 365*, we will cover the three main components of a diet, which will provide plenty of fruits, vegetables, and whole grains that include common superfoods, and combine them with good healthy fats and lean protein. The meal plans will also help you keep a healthy gut by including probiotic and prebiotic foods in your diet.

When people embark on a new diet or begin to eat healthy, they think that it has to be boring. I always say that eating healthy doesn't have to be boring or daunting. You can actually apply these principles and have delicious, easy meals. A lot of people also think that eating healthy foods needs to come in the form of a smoothie. With this book and the resource material available to you on www.flatbelly.com/resources, I will show you how to include these powerful foods in various ways from soups and grain bowls to salads, smoothies, and much more. At the same time, these meal plans vary, not just in season, but also in temperature, so you can have a warm Cannellini Chicken Sausage bowl (see page 118) in the winter to a California Avocado Gazpacho (see page 73) in the summer. Eating can be fun, eating can be exciting, and it can be a love relationship with your taste buds and your gut.

I am honored and excited to introduce the *Flat-Belly 365* plan and educate you about how to reduce your belly fat by enjoying exquisite recipes using superfoods. My clients' successes have been my passion and inspiration and continue to be so. This diet is not a gimmick or a new trend. This is a way of living that has been proven through solid research and will provide lasting results.

I look forward to sharing my wisdom and culinary skills with you in *Flat-Belly 365*. This plan is a delicious way to lose weight that will last a lifetime. Expect to reboot your gut, improve your total health, and have more energy than you have felt in years. Get ready to experience a lifelong journey of superfoods that will keep you strong, healthy, and rejuvenated.

CHAPTER 1

The Secret to Success: Gut-Friendly Superfoods

All Body Fat Is Not Created Equal

When losing weight, it is important to consider the types of body fat that we have. Not all body fat is created equal. There are 2 main types of fat in our bodies: some of these fats can be harmful to health in large amounts, and others can actually be beneficial. It is also important to know that where this fat is located in your body can have an impact on your health.

Subcutaneous Fat

This is the type of fat found directly under the skin, specifically between the skin in the muscle. This type of fat cells, when weight is gained, increases in number, not in size. This fat is also found throughout your entire body. This includes the arms, legs, buttocks, and belly. However, not all of this fat is bad, depending on the location. Many studies have shown that those with a higher distribution of fat around the thighs and buttocks could be at a lower risk of heart disease. Studies also suggest that the fats in these areas get encapsulated so that fats do not harm the other organs. For many people, having excess subcutaneous fat is a concern for appearance reasons.

Visceral Fat

The worst fat that a person can have is visceral fat. Visceral fat is inflammatory and surrounds your organs. This is also called "deep fat" or "abdominal fat" and is in an area that lies out of reach, so it cannot be easily pinched or felt like subcutaneous fat. In fact, this fat is the culprit of many chronic diseases, such as hypertension, metabolic syndrome, diabetes, cardiovascular disease, and even certain cancers. When someone gains weight, visceral fat cells grow in size, not in number. When they get to be too large, it becomes toxic and begins to constantly produce inflammatory chemicals called cytokines, which lead to inflammation. At the same time, these cytokines interfere with hormones that regulate appetite, mood, and brain function.

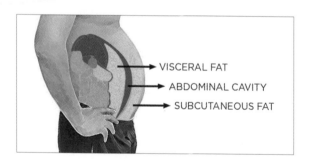

Your Belly Fat

Your belly fat is composed of subcutaneous fat and visceral fat. We all are supposed to have these types of fats in our belly for protection of the internal organs. However, when in excess it is detrimental to your health. If a man's waistline is bigger than 40 inches and a woman's is greater than 35 inches, they are at risk of chronic inflammation.

Chronic Inflammation

There are two types of inflammation that your body experiences: acute and chronic. Acute inflammation is the type of inflammation that happens when you get a cut and it becomes red and tender, or "inflamed." This is a normal and beneficial response from your immune system for healing. It is temporary and eventually goes away.

Chronic inflammation, however, is a completely different story. Chronic inflammation is when your immune response is turned on, but it doesn't shut off. You can't see or feel it and it's difficult to test for. Your body is constantly releasing inflammatory chemicals, such as cytokines, that are produced from factors such as having excess visceral fat. This is a systemic condition in which cells, artery walls, and fibers are affected, which leads to other chronic diseases and advanced aging. Chronic inflammation can also be caused by lifestyle factors, such as smoking, alcohol, and lack of sleep.

Lastly, your diet alone, even without excess visceral fat, can cause inflammation. High-fat fried foods, processed foods, excess sugar, and refined carbs have been known to contribute to chronic inflammation. The good news is that you can markedly decrease inflammation in your body by losing your belly fat and eating anti-inflammatory superfoods, such as blueberries, broccoli, chia seeds, salmon, and avocados, among others.

Eat Fat to Lose Fat

First let me tell you that the only way to lose visceral fat is through diet and exercise alone. It is important to understand what foods to eat, especially which fats. Your body reacts differently depending on the kind of fat you eat. A diet that is high in saturated fat and processed foods builds more belly fat. However, certain fats can help reduce visceral fat. This is where monounsaturated and omega-3 fats come into play. Monounsaturated fats are good anti-inflammatory fats found in plant-based foods and have a host of amazing health benefits, including a decreased risk of breast cancer, lower cholesterol levels, a lower risk of heart disease, and, most important, there is sufficient evidence that shows that monounsaturated fat decreases belly fat. Monounsaturated fats can be found in canola and olive oil, avocados, almonds, and walnuts, among other foods.

Omega-3 fats are another type of potent anti-inflammatory and beneficial fat found in plant and animal sources. Omega-3 fats have been shown to help the body break down visceral fat. Animal sources are mainly fish, such as sardines and salmon, and plant-based sources are walnuts, flax seeds, and chia seeds.

Be aware that even though these two fats help reduce belly fat, you still need to eat them in the proper portions. Eating too much fat of any kind increases your calorie intake and could lead to weight gain. But no worries, I have taken all of this into consideration in developing the meal plans for *Flat-Belly 365*.

Eat Antioxidant and Anti-Inflammatory Foods

Free radicals are a real problem. A free radical is an unstable molecule that latches onto healthy cells and makes them unstable, which then creates a chain reaction. They are created by your environment, diet, smoking, alcohol, and visceral fat, among other factors. Their number one characteristic is their ability to react with our DNA and mutate the strains. As we know, mutated genes can lead to cancer or other diseases, and the chronic inflammation caused by these free radicals is almost as bad.

I can't say this enough: The key to healthy nutrition is variety. The way to help your body repair and restore itself and to improve your overall health is through a full range of colorful superfoods. Superfoods are not just limited to fruits and vegetables but also include grains such as black rice, quinoa, and legumes. Phytochemicals that give plants their color have antioxidant effects. The antioxidants in anti-inflammatory fruits, vegetables, herbs, whole grains, and fats not only can help reduce the effects of the inflammation created by visceral fat but also can help reduce the number and effect of free radicals by neutralizing free-floating free radicals throughout the body. Because each phytochemical has different strengths, you need to eat a rainbow of them, not just one.

Anthocyanins, for instance, provide the purple in blueberries, some raspberries, and purple potatoes. They have powerful antioxidant effects. Carotene, which gives carrots and orange melons their color, has also been shown to preserve cognitive function as we age. Lycopene, which makes tomatoes red, has been shown to reduce the risk of prostate cancer in men. These effects are also cumulative, since no single food is a magic bullet. These healthy pigments, together, can provide support for your body. You want the full diversity of the rainbow.

Eat to Build Your Right Microbiome

If all that wasn't enough, here is the last punch line. We should all take a look at the gut, the forgotten organ. The gut microbiome significantly affects human health and disease. The majority of these gut microbes are located in the colon and affect the immune system, inflammation, digestion, weight gain, and much more. Each individual has a unique microbial composition, just like a fingerprint, which is determined by many factors: stress, intestinal infections, poor hygiene, smoking, alcohol, medications, and, most importantly, your diet.

There have been talks and debates recently about the different types of bacteria living within our bodies. Researchers have only begun to scratch the surface of this field, yet many studies are already linking migraines, low immunity, depression, type 2 diabetes, heart disease, gastrointestinal disorders, low energy, and even weight gain to bacteria in the gastrointestinal tract.

In our gastrointestinal tract, there are over 1,000 separate bacterial species that can reach a total number in the tens of billions. Not all of these bacteria are bad. Most of them are the "good" or "helpful" type of bacteria, also known as probiotics. So, what are probiotics? They are live, acting organisms that help keep the digestive system in happy and healthy.

The food you eat affects the composition of your microbiome. A poor diet that is low in fiber allows the bad bacteria in our guts to grow and multiply. Therefore, your goal is to limit your intake of high sugar, high fat, fried foods, and highly refined carbohydrates because bad bacteria can trigger weight gain.

Your Gut Bacteria Can Make You Fat

Having a healthy gut with the right balance of good bacteria can change the entire health of our bodies. Studies have shown that the right combination of gut bacteria can cause changes in a person's weight. There is growing evidence of a connection between gut microbiome and the role that it may play in weight loss. Researchers have even identified the probiotic species and strains of bacteria that can help decrease body fat, such as those in the Lactobacillus family.

Researchers can now identify an individual as obese or lean just by looking at their gut bacteria. Several studies have transplanted microbes from obese mice into lean mice, which resulted in weight and fat gain without any changes in their diet and exercise. The same result occurred when the microbiome of lean mice was transplanted into obese mice; they lost weight. One explanation for this is that the bad bacteria slows down both the transit of food in the intestines and the extraction of more calories, resulting in weight gain. This could be happening to humans as well.

The 5 Gut-Healthy Principles

Principle 1—Eat Probiotics

Yes, you can eat these good bacteria, especially Lactobacillus and bifidobacterium, which have been linked to various health benefits. These types of living bacteria are found naturally in food, especially in fermented dairy products such as yogurts, aged cheeses, and kefir. They are also found in non-dairy foods such as tofu, natto, and tempeh. A great way to start adding probiotics to your diet is to begin your day with a breakfast smoothie made with yogurt or kefir, snack on a chunk of Parmesan cheese paired with an apple, and switch your chicken stir-fry night to tempeh stir-fry.

Principle 2—Eat Fermented Foods

The fermentation process of vegetables enables the growth of the probiotics lactobacillus and bifidobacterium. Therefore, adding fermented vegetables to your diet will not only increase your probiotics, but also your vegetable intake. This is also a great way for vegans or people with lactose intolerance to get probiotics. Fermented vegetable products such as pickles, sauerkraut, kimchi, and kombucha are great sources of probiotics. For this reason, I recommend that part of your vegetable count be fermented. Fermenting vegetables is super easy to do, and once fermented, they can last in the refrigerator for weeks. Check out my fermented vegetable recipe on page 130 or visit *www.flatbelly365.com/resources* for a tutorial video to learn a quick and easy way to make your own fermented vegetables.

If you don't want to make your own, fermented vegetables are easy to find at your local supermarkets, but make sure they are fermented with sea salt and without vinegar. Ionized salt and vinegar will prevent the fermentation process that is necessary for the good bacteria to flourish. More than likely, these fermented vegetables will be found in the refrigerator section of your grocery.

Principle 3—Eat Prebiotics

As humans, we need food to function. And just like us, probiotics need fuel to function and, most important, to multiply. This is where prebiotics come into play. Prebiotics are nondigestible fibers found in good carbohydrate foods, such as whole grains, legumes, fruits, and vegetables. However, not all fibers are created equal. Prebiotics must meet certain criteria. These fibers must be resistant to digestion and be able to be fermented by bacteria in the intestine. There are many types of prebiotic fibers, including fructo-oligosaccharides (FOS), inulin, oligofructose, and galacto-oligosaccardes (GOS), which are found specifically in asparagus, Jerusalem artichokes, leeks, jicama, onions, garlic, chicory root, yams, avocado, bananas, apples, oats, and barley, among others. So make a delicious oatmeal with applesauce topped with sliced bananas or snack on jicama with lime juice and chili powder.

Resistant starch is another type of complex carbohydrate that doesn't get digested in the small intestine but rather in the colon and acts as a prebiotic. When this starch is fermented in the colon by gut bacteria, it produces short chain fatty acids (SCFAs) like butyrate. Butyrate is good for gut bacteria and known to be anti-inflammatory. Good sources of resistant starch are lentils, green peas, uncooked rolled oats, green bananas, and white beans.

Also, the type of fat you eat can increase the diversity of the gut microbiome and weight. A recent study done with walnuts shows a positive effect on the gut bacteria by increasing good bacteria, Lactobacillus, Ruminococcaceae, and

Roseburia and decreasing bad bacteria. One of the mechanisms suggested that this is due to the effect of the walnuts' significant amount of alpha-linolenic acid (ALA), the plant-based omega-3 fatty acid (2.5 grams per one ounce), and fiber. In this way, walnuts are acting as a prebiotic.

Principle 4—Fiber Up

Fiber has always been good for your gut and health regardless of whether you eat probiotics or prebiotics. Making sure we consume soluble and insoluble fibers is key for good health and weight control. Soluble fiber is one of the foods that can help control your hunger by making you satisfied for longer periods of time, and therefore you eat less. Soluble fiber is found in apples, oatmeal, beans, barley, and Brussels sprouts, among other foods. Insoluble fiber "cleans you up" and makes you regular, resulting in a healthy gut. These fibers are found in fruits, vegetables, and whole grains, so go at it!

Principle 5—Clean Up

It's understood that smoking, stress, alcohol, and antibiotic intake can affect your gut balance. It is not difficult to change the balance of your gut bacteria and create conditions that are conducive to bad bacteria. Therefore, limit or avoid smoking and alcohol intake, manage stress, and try to limit antibiotic intake as much as possible.

With the Flat-Belly 365 Plan, I have put together all the science that is mentioned above and combined it to provide an effective way for you to achieve your health goals. This program is designed to provide plenty of superfoods that are full of antioxidants and vitamins and minerals that are good for a healthy metabolism and for general health. The plan also provides the right amount of anti-inflammatory fats and prebiotic and probiotic foods that will not only help you lose belly fat, but also make you feel young and energized.

Table 1: Prebiotic and Probiotic Foods*

Prebiotic	Probiotic
Onions	Yogurt
Tomatoes	Kefir
Asparagus	Coconut kefir
Jerusalem artichokes	Aged cheese
Leeks	Fermented vegetables
Jicama	Sauerkraut
Garlic	Kimchi
Yams	Kombucha
Bananas	Tempeh
Avocado	Fermented Tofu
Chicory root	Natto
Prunes	Miso
Dandelion greens	Wheat-free tamari
Barley	Traditional buttermilk
Oats	
Quinoa	

For a downloadable version of this table, visit www.flatbelly365.com/resources

CHAPTER 2

The Flat-Belly 365 Plan

Starting a new program can be confusing and overwhelming. We are so accustomed to our normal habits and day-to-day routines that the thought of altering our lifestyle is daunting. You may feel stuck because you don't know how to begin. You may feel tempted by bagels at work on Wednesdays or Doughnut Fridays. You may suffer from the Weekend Warrior syndrome, where you are good all week long and then blow it during the weekend fiestas. You are in a rut and don't know how to break the cycle. Therefore, your intentions to get healthy are put off for another day.

Not to mention that there is a constant stream of misleading information out there suggesting to "Eat this" or "Eat that" for fast weight loss or some other health benefit. Some articles even suggest different times of day to eat certain types of food to increase their health benefits. With all this information, it can become overwhelming to not only start but to know where to start. This is why I created Flat-Belly 365 meal plans that include all my latest findings in nutrition and food and how to put them together. The thinking is done for you; all you need to do is follow the plan.

The first seven days will be considered your reboot week, giving your body a chance for your body to function optimally. This week is meant to refresh and rebalance your internal organs. You will replenish yourself with nutrients, rejuvenate your system, and improve your health. This week will get you off your vicious cycle and start the process of rebuilding your gut flora, reducing abdominal fat, and fighting inflammation to achieve a flat belly.

This reboot week can be used any time of the year when you need a quick boost. For example, when you come home after a long vacation or a big holiday weekend, you may feel sluggish or out of sync. Maybe you drank too much alcohol or you ate too many sugary treats. Perhaps you ate your way through the holidays, and your clothes are squeezing the breath out of you. You suddenly notice a muffin top when wearing your skinny jeans. Now is the time to refresh, rejuvenate, and restore your health. Throughout this week, you will get your balance back, realign your hormones, cleanse your internal organs, increase your energy, improve your skin, optimize your vitality, and lose those extra pounds you gained.

This week will begin your journey toward establishing new habits, such as menu planning, shopping, and preparing healthy meals and snacks. By taking time for yourself and prioritizing your nutrition goals, you will set a foundation for long-term successful habits. By the end of the week, you will be motivated to continue eating delicious, nutritious foods in the days to come.

How the Plan Works

Each chapter is separated and organized by the different seasons of the year: spring, summer, fall, and winter. Within each chapter, you will find a 7-Day Flat-Belly plan that presents a combination of recipes and snacks to keep you full throughout the day. Each recipe and snack is also based on the seasonality of fruits and vegetables. Given that California produces a significant majority of the fruits, vegetables, and nuts sold in the United States, I decided to follow California's seasonal growing chart, which focuses on American-grown superfoods such as almonds, walnuts, strawberries, blueberries, avocado, and broccoli, among many others. Take note that no matter what state you live in, you will have access to this seasonal produce. If for some reason your state doesn't follow California's seasonality, you will still be able to get the produce from a foreign country, which is fine. For example, blueberries grow in California in the summer months, which means you're most likely eating California blueberries during those months. However, during fall, the blueberries you're eating may be from another country, such as Chile.

Within each season, the recipes have a variety of textures and temperatures designed to reflect the rich abundance of foods, as well as the changing climate. For example, during the summer months, we have a variety of gazpachos, light, refreshing salads, and cold smoothies for hot days. During the cold winter months, we incorporate hot, heartier soups, grain bowls, and warm smoothies. This lends a more satisfying experience with each meal. The plan is customizable to you—you can choose your meals and snacks from any season you wish.

Meal Plans for Men and Women

The menus are also divided up by 1,300 calories and 1,800 calories, which are both designed to achieve a flat belly. For women, I have chosen a caloric range of 1,300 calories. This plan was developed for females who are 20 to 59 years old, with an average lifestyle that includes a desk job. During the flat belly phase, we recommend weekly exercises. Refer to the Flat-Belly 365 Exercise plan (page 32) for specific recommendations. For women older than 60 years old who exercise three times or less per week, you will need to cut your calories by 100 per day to successfully lose weight. As we age gracefully, our metabolisms naturally decrease. Therefore, by eliminating one snack every day from the sample menus, you can cut an extra 100 calories for optimal weight loss. Another option is to adjust your lunch or dinner by reducing your portion size slightly. For example, eat 50 calories less at lunch and at dinner. Simply cut 50 calories by reducing your carbohydrate intake by half.

For men, I have chosen a caloric range of 1,800 calories to achieve a flat belly. This plan was developed for males who are 20 to 59 years old, with an average lifestyle that includes a desk job. During the flat belly phase, we recommend weekly exercises. Refer to the Flat Belly 365 Exercise plan (page 32) for specific recommendations. If you need a bit more than 1,800 calories, just add another snack to your day or increase your portion sizes by another ½ cup for each meal.

For a Flat Belly, Count Food, Not Calories

You've noticed that I talk about a caloric range for women and men, 1,300 and 1,800 respectively. You may be wondering why you can't just count calories. This question often pops up in my private practice when clients inevitably ask me: "Why are you talking about calories when you don't want me to count calories?" Calories, contrary to popular belief, are not all the same. Unfortunately, this perpetuates the idea that calories are the single most important component of a person's diet. While every calorie may provide the same amount of energy, they do, in fact, differ quite a bit. Frankly, at the end of the day, calories do count, but where they come from may cause significant differences in terms of weight loss and overall health.

What is vital to remember when trying to achieve a flat belly is that you are consuming less food than your body is burning, which is the simple science of weight loss. However, when you do this, you put yourself at risk of not getting enough nutrients, because you are focusing only on counting calories. It is important to know where your calories are coming from and what they are providing you. Calories that lack enough micronutrients such as vitamins, minerals, and phytonutrients can ultimately slow your metabolism because many of these micronutrients play a role in maintaining an efficient metabolism.

To further illustrate the difference between counting calories or not, let's think about two types of grains. A cup of white rice and a cup of quinoa have roughly the same calorie content of 210. However, the two foods differ with respect to micronutrient makeup because quinoa has a vitamin, mineral, and phytonutrient content that white rice fails to offer. Indeed, you can lose weight with both types of grains, but given that quinoa has more micronutrients, in the long run, it can promote better weight loss because its micronutrients help to fuel an efficient metabolism. In addition, quinoa contains fiber and protein that can help keep you fuller longer. Protein and fiber are nutrients that have been proven to promote satiety the longest due to their long digestive processes. Simple carbohydrates digest quickly and cause you to be hungry again sooner.

Also, those who count calories may not pay close attention to the composition of their meals and, in so doing, may create hormonal spikes that stall weight loss over time. This may not apply to all, but definitely does to those who are experiencing insulin resistance, which is likely with larger waistlines. The composition of your meal is important because your metabolic hormones will respond differently to different macronutrients, and may even create a vicious cycle. A meal that is high in simple carbohydrates like white rice will spike up your insulin in response to the rising levels of glucose in your blood. However, because your body is experiencing insulin resistance, your insulin levels will stay elevated longer, which creates a vicious cycle because the insulin will store fat around your waistline, which generates more insulin resistance.

As you can see, calories are not all equal when it comes to weight loss and health. Counting calories can slow down your metabolism, make you hungry, disrupt your hormones, and cause you to lose muscle. You can have your pleasurable foods, but be mindful of the quality of the calories you are consuming and try to eat a balance of good sources of carbohydrates, lean proteins, and healthy fats. In this book, I provide meal plans that will take away the calorie counting task and give you a balanced, lifestyle approach to weight loss.

How to Be Successful

Shopping

First things first: the most important thing to do is have the right food available in your home. People always have great intentions to start a program, but if the right food is not in the house, efforts get derailed. For this reason, I have developed a shopping list for each of the seasons to make things a bit easier for you. Before you head over to the grocery store or farmers' market, be sure to revise the shopping list to map out where you need to go or what ingredients you might need. Also, these shopping lists include ingredients that are needed for only the recipes in each of the 7-day menu plans. If you choose to replace one recipe with another, please be sure to look at the recipe and buy the proper ingredients. Other things to consider are basic cooking utensils, knives, a cutting board, pots, pans, a blender, mixing bowls, and measuring cups and spoons. Also, storage containers are important. Be sure to have large and small containers to store or transport your soups, cooked whole grains, and salads.

Cooking

Give yourself enough time and space to cook for your week. Cook one day out of the weekend, or a different day when you are completely commitment free, and prepare meals with longer cooking times such as soups, dressings, and selected grain bowls. On average, most people take only about 3 to 4 hours to shop and cook. Once the shopping and cooking are done, the rest of the days of the week are assembly days. Some of the salads or smoothie bowls can be made the day of or the night before.

Stay within the Portions

These meal plans were designed with specific caloric recommendations and macronutrient percentages to achieve a flat belly. If you choose to substitute one meal for another, please feel free, but make sure you stay within the portion sizes for fruits, grains, nuts, seeds, oil, and dressings.

Variation

The majority of the recipes were created as four servings so that they could be used multiple times throughout the week. As you will see in the 7-day flat belly plans, recipes are used multiple times during a week, in an alternating manner. This allows for variation, giving you the opportunity to mix up the order and prevent boredom. For example, you can have soup for 2 days, and then you can include a salad or a grain bowl as a third meal. If you prefer to eat the same salad or soup for 5 consecutive days, that is okay, too. The best part about the menus is that you have options. If there is a recipe you are not interested in making, don't make it. Simply use another recipe from another day of the week. All the recipes provide about the same number of calories per meal, so swapping one recipe for another is completely acceptable and encouraged.

Watch Your Snacks

I've provided you with two snacks a day. If you're not hungry, you don't need to eat every single snack. The snacks are suggested in order to control hunger levels and ensure optimal energy and brain function. The main goal is to stay fueled. By eating every 3 to 4 hours, you will control ghrelin levels, which is the hunger hormone. Ghrelin spikes when we wait more than 3 hours between meals or skip them. Research tells us that eating every 3 hours is about the right interval to manage ghrelin, which controls both hunger and appetite.

For example, within 30 minutes after a meal, ghrelin begins to rise steadily until the next meal. Studies have shown that a longer break between meals is associated with a more significant increase in ghrelin production. Studies have also demonstrated that there is less ghrelin produced in the average person between breakfast and lunch (a 3- to 4-hour break) than between lunch and dinner (typically 6 hours), so timing the space between meals is a critical modulator of ghrelin. With this knowledge, you may not need a snack between breakfast and lunch. But you will definitely need a snack between lunch and dinner. This is super important for controlling your hunger.

Ghrelin spikes when we lose weight. Why? Because your body only cares about survival. It wants homeostasis, or the status quo. Your body thinks losing weight is dangerous, so as you start to lose, you need to be extra mindful of your ghrelin function. Your body will fight back if you don't approach weight loss in a steady, sensible way, working with your ghrelin instead of against it. This is a fundamental principle to understand: you have to eat regularly to lose weight. Two problems that occur during weight loss are consuming too few calories at each meal or avoiding carbohydrates. You will not have to worry about these challenges. Every meal provides you with a well-balanced mix of healthy carbohydrates, proteins, and fats, in addition to adequate calorie intake.

If you still remain hungry after your snacks, add more fermented vegetables or plain raw vegetables.

Vegetarians and Vegans

Please note, the base for the majority of these recipes is either vegan or vegetarian. If there is a recipe in the meal plan that does not follow your dietary preference, simply replace it with a vegan recipe. Make sure you still use the proper amount of protein. See Table 2 for vegan protein options. Another recommendation to meet your protein requirement is to have a protein shake with your meal. For example, if you are a vegan, you can have the Wild Rice with Stir Fry Vegetable Bowl (see page 98) alongside a protein shake made with either rice or pea protein with 4 fluid ounces of almond milk or water. Be sure to have 16 grams of protein in your shake if you are female or 30 grams if you are male.

Protein Options

All meal plans are based on using grilled or baked chicken breast as the protein source. To add variation, we have provided you with a chart of other lean protein options. Table 2 lists the proper amounts of different proteins.

Table 2: Protein Sources*

This table illustrates the proper amount, in ounces, of the different types of proteins that can be used with each 7-day flat belly plan. Please keep in mind that some of these protein sources are also a fat source and have a higher caloric level for the same amount of protein provided. Visit Chapter 7 on page 129 to see some delicious ways to cook your protein choices.

Amount	Protein Sources	Calories	Protein (g)
3 ounces	Chicken breast	128	22
3 ounces	Pork loin	178	20
3 ounces	Sirloin	156	24
3 ounces	Lamb (leg loin, leg, rack)	150	23
3 ounces	White fish	111	22
3 ounces	Tuna, canned	70	16
3 ounces	Salmon	155	21
3 ounces	Shrimp	84	20
2 each	Whole egg	156	14
6 each	Egg whites	91	20.5
5 ounces	Tofu, extra firm	117	20
3 ounces	Seitan	120	21
3 ounces	Tempeh	167	19

* For a downloadable version of this table, visit www.flatbelly365.com/resources

Topping options

Toppings are included in some of the recipes. In the 7-day flat belly plans, smoothie bowls, breakfast grain bowls, or yogurts are used for breakfasts or snacks. These recipes call for certain toppings; if you decide to change the toppings, be sure to keep the same amounts as indicated in the menus. Table 3 lists the proper amounts of different toppings.

Table 3: Toppings*

This table sets forth the different toppings that can be used in the smoothie bowl, breakfast grain bowl, and yogurt recipes. Each of these serving provides about **50 calories**. Please adjust accordingly based on your calorie levels.

Fruit	Nuts and Seeds	Others
¾ blueberries	1 tablespoon sunflower seeds	2 tablespoons dry oats
¾ cup strawberries	1 tablespoon chia seeds	¼ cup popped amaranth
¾ cup raspberries	1 tablespoon anise seeds	1 tablespoon cacao nibs
¾ cup blackberries	1 tablespoon pumpkin seeds	1 tablespoon unsweetened coconut flakes
¾ cup fresh pichuberries	1 tablespoon whole flaxseed	1 tablespoon granola
4 tablespoons pomegranate seeds	1 tablespoon hemp seeds	1 tablespoon buckwheat groats
2 tablespoons dried cranberries	6 almonds	1 tablespoon bee pollen
2 tablespoons dried pichuberries	6 cashews	
2 tablespoons raisins	15 pistachios	
1 tablespoon dried goji berries	1 tablespoon chopped walnuts	
2 prunes	1 tablespoon pecans	

For a downloadable version of this table, visit www.flatbelly365.com/resources

Coffee and Tea

Coffee and green tea are allowed during the first seven days, but you should refrain from creamers and all sugars. Both beverages provide antioxidants as well as other benefits, including immune-boosting abilities, cardiovascular health, and memory function. Studies have shown that aside from providing energy, coffee is packed with antioxidants that can help reduce the risk of type 2 diabetes, improve memory, and benefit cardiovascular health.

But how many cups do you really need? All these studies suggest that the right amount of coffee is between 2 to 3 cups a day. Aha! Moderation again is the answer. Remember, 1 cup is 8 fluid ounces.

Green tea is a great fluid to help keep you hydrated. If you are worried about the caffeine content, consider looking into decaf options. For the first 7 days, refrain from adding creamer or sugar, as both of these not only add more calories, but also counteract the health benefits of coffee and green tea.

Alcohol Intake

Refrain from drinking alcoholic beverages during your first 7 days. This will allow you to see maximum results. Following the first week, you can reintroduce alcohol. Drinking alcohol is definitely a choice that only you can make. Moderation is important, so if you do drink alcohol, it can be worked into your plan. Take note: When your liver is processing alcohol, it cannot process fat—it only does one function at a time. So, the fact that you're not metabolizing fat when you're drinking means you're holding on to the fats that would otherwise be processed. If you drink, this doesn't mean you need to stop drinking. It only means that drinking too much too often may slow or even stop your fat loss. To be successful, follow the tips below:

Tips for alcohol consumption:

1) Think of a drink as a special occasion situation and not a daily habit.
2) Consume no more than four to six servings of alcohol per week for ideal weight loss and a flat belly.

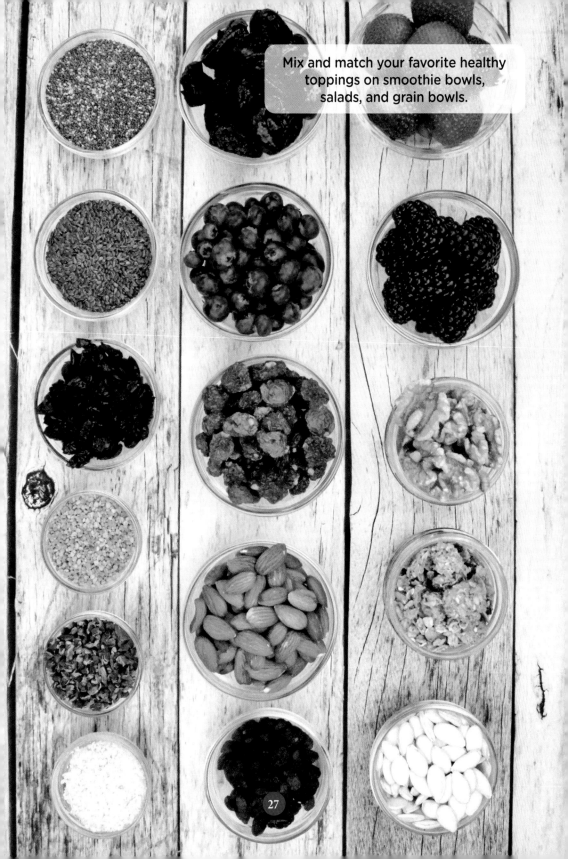

Mix and match your favorite healthy toppings on smoothie bowls, salads, and grain bowls.

27

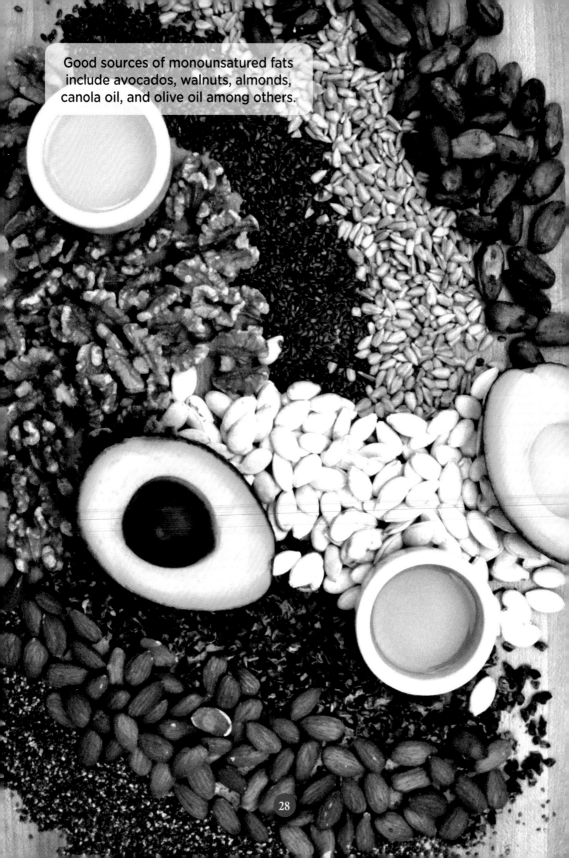

Good sources of monounsatured fats include avocados, walnuts, almonds, canola oil, and olive oil among others.

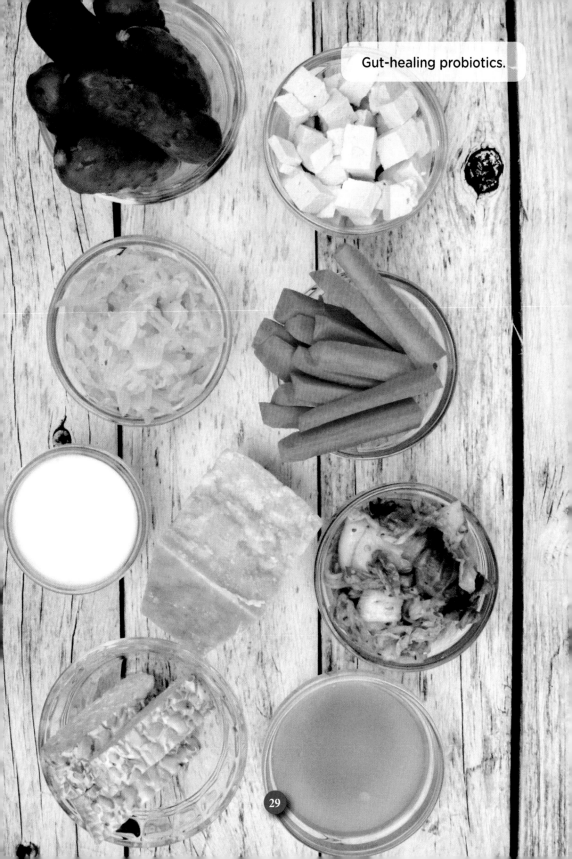

Gut-healing probiotics.

Ferment your own vegetables or
buy them at your local grocery store.
See the recipe on page 130.

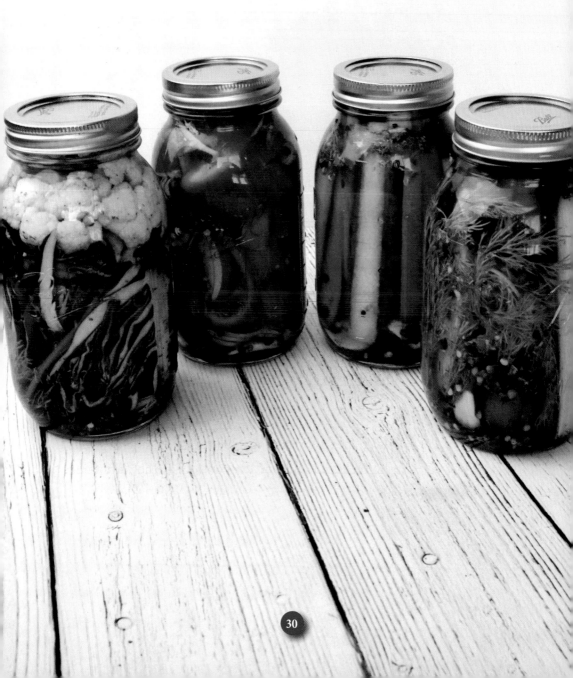

3) For a flat belly, although there's no specific research, observations suggest that men may have 6 servings per week, while women may have four servings per week.

4) Serving sizes: 1 serving of alcohol is equivalent to 4 ounces of wine, a shot of booze (1.5 ounces), or 12 ounces of beer.

5) The oversized globe wineglasses in restaurants contain 6 ounces a pour (one and a half servings). A glass of wine in your house usually equals 8 ounces (two servings). Cocktails in restaurants may include 2 shots and equal 2 servings.

6) Alcohol stimulates appetite, which puts you at risk for higher calorie intake. Alcohol also lowers your inhibitions, making it easier to choose unhealthy foods.

7) Many people enjoy a glass of wine with dinner as a matter of course, or because they are foodies. Instead of wine at every dinner, enjoy it when you're at restaurants on weekends, or once a week, not every day. Remember that, when you are drinking alcohol, your body is not metabolizing fat, which is counter to your weight loss efforts.

Sweets

Refrain from consuming sweets for the first 7 days. This will allow you to see maximum results. Following the first week, you can reintroduce sweets. Sweets are treats and need to be regulated and portion controlled. There's nothing wrong with wanting to finish a meal with a sweet delicacy. Fighting your sweet tooth can cause problems of bingeing or overconsumption. Make the recipes. Enjoy the right portion for you and experience the love as needed. If you decide to add dessert to your meal plans, keep in mind the total calories for the day as indicated on page 17.

A few of my favorite suggestions with full antioxidants are:

1) Two tablets of dark chocolate paired with two dried figs
2) Two dates filled with 1 tablespoon of cacao nibs
3) 1 cup of strawberries topped with vanilla yogurt
4) 100 percent fruit popsicles, especially mango; simply puree mango chunks and some lime juice, freeze, and enjoy
5) Grilled pineapples
6) Baked Apples with Cinnamon and Chia (see page 145)
7) Citrus Raspberry Chia Seed Pudding (see page 144)

Flat-Belly 365 Exercise

For an optimal flat belly, which means losing fat and maintaining lean muscle mass, your weight loss efforts should be 80 percent nutrition and 20 percent exercise. This is the 80/20 Rule. I am a fierce advocate for exercising for health. However, exercise is not the primary means to obtain a flat belly or even to lose weight. It's not about how much you exercise for a flat belly. It's about how much you eat for a flat belly. Be as active as you can be, but remember that what you put in your mouth is what will speed up or inhibit your flat belly. Here are the guidelines for exercise.

Low-Intensity Flat-Belly Exercise

Examples: walking, hatha yoga, stretching, easy swimming, lightweight training, bicycling less than 10 mph, golfing using a cart, light yard work or housework

Needs: The meal plans provide you with two daily snacks. Make sure to have a snack before the workout. This is all you need for fuel, regardless of how many times a week you work out at a low intensity.

High-Intensity Flat-Belly Exercise

Examples: circuit training, CrossFit, boot camps, high-intensity body-pumping classes, spinning, running for 45 minutes or more, boxing, kickboxing, intense swimming, vigorous dance classes

Needs: People who exercise at a high intensity should include the extra pre-workout flat-belly shake (the shake is not shown in the sample meal plans). If you are working out, drink the shake 45 minutes to 1 hour prior to the activity. Stay fueled and do not create a bigger deficit between energy expended and energy consumed. Losing fat is not about deprivation and eating little amounts of food. You want to stay powered and energized so you can blast the belly fat, reboot your body, and get that waistline you've always wanted.

Flat-Belly Pre-Exercise Shake

Female Pre-Exercise Shake	Male Pre-Exercise Shake
1 medium banana, 5 to 6 inches	1 medium banana, 7 to 8 inches
2 teaspoons maca** powder (optional) 1 tablespoon cacao powder	1 tablespoon maca** powder (optional) 1 tablespoon cacao powder
1 cup milk of choice (cow, rice, almond, soy)	1 cup milk of choice (cow, rice, almond, soy)
15–20g of protein powder of choice (whey, rice, pea, or soy)	20–25g of protein powder of choice (whey, rice, pea, or soy)

** *Maca is a native Peruvian superfood root that grows in the Andes and resembles a small rough stone the size of a walnut. Maca has a positive effect on energy and mood. As studies have shown, it can support continued exercise because it increases glucose in the blood stream. While rich in amino acids, phytonutrients, and a variety of vitamins and minerals, maca functions as an adaptogen, thus aiding in adrenal function to increase energy, reduce stress, and create an overall revitalizing effect. I usually take maca in my pre-exercise shake.*

Directions

1) Put all the ingredients in a blender and puree until the shake is the desired consistency.

To feel the effects of maca, you need to consume the shake four to five times per week, not just once a week or on a sporadic basis. Enjoy the shake 45 minutes to one hour before the workout.

Cravings Cheat Sheet

Craving salt—instead, try fermented vegetables like kimchi, pickles, sauerkraut, cauliflower, or carrots. These are all great sources of probiotics, too (See page 14).

Craving sugar—instead, chew on 2 tablespoons cacao nibs (only once per day).

Craving alcohol—instead, drink sparkling water with a lime for a fabulous mocktail.

Craving food—instead of suffering from hunger and ruining your metabolism, make sure to have your snacks. You can munch on nonstarchy vegetables without dealing with any guilt. This includes broccoli, tomato, carrots, bell peppers, or any other vegetable that you love. Check each chapter for more detailed examples.

---

6 Flat-Belly 365 Principles

Flat-Belly Must-Do #1

Eat breakfast within 90 minutes of waking. Be sure your breakfast is a blend of carbohydrates, fiber, and protein. My plan offers many recipes that satisfy this principle. Breakfast is the most important meal, and it drives your entire day. It determines how much you're going to eat at 4:00 p.m. Breakfast will control your hunger hormone ghrelin and set you up for success. If you exercise in the morning, have a pre-exercise shake (see the Flat-Belly Pre-Exercise Shake recipe on page 33) and then breakfast after the workout. Having the shake before the workout will increase your metabolism, boost your performance, help with clear thinking, improve alertness and concentration, enhance memory, and improve cognitive abilities for the entire day.

Flat-Belly Must-Do #2

Do not skip meals. There is a lot of contradictory research about mealtimes. Some people say you should eat 3 meals a day, while others say you should eat 5 or 6. For many people, 3 square meals don't work anymore. These days, many of us wake up at 5:00 a.m. and stay up until midnight. Plus, we work harder and expend more brain power, which uses up fuel. You need to eat every 3 to 4 hours to control ghrelin, so depending on how many waking hours you have, you may need 4 meals or you may need 6.

Flat-Belly Must-Do #3

At every main meal, combine carbohydrates, proteins, and fats. This gives you the optimal blend of nutritional elements to fight cravings, control hunger, and gain energy. Protein increases your metabolism while carbs lower ghrelin, help with brain function, and decrease cravings. Fat provides satiety. Every meal in the sample menus provides this optimum combination.

It doesn't matter what time you stop eating. It is a myth that we shouldn't eat after a certain time in the evening. Just give yourself at least 90 minutes before you plan to go to sleep. You need those 90 minutes to digest so you can sleep comfortably. I like to think of this as the 70/30 Rule, which means you should eat 70 percent of your calories before dinnertime and 30 percent at dinner, whatever time that may be.

Flat-Belly Must-Do #4

Stay hydrated. You've heard it a million times, but drinking water is essential for keeping energy up, aiding metabolism, burning fat, and more. It's the fluid your body needs for life, and it's an instrumental part in your weight loss. Other fluids can be useful, but water is the best choice because it is calorie free. Forget about that whole 8 cups a day thing. I want you to relax and remember to have a healthy amount of water whenever you think of it. Thirst can confuse your sense of hunger, so make sure you stay hydrated. Try infusing your water by adding pineapple or kiwi slices to it to provide some flavor. Make sure you throw out the pineapple or kiwi after 2 days and replenish it with a new batch to maintain optimal freshness.

Flat-Belly Must-Do #5

De-stressed to get a flat belly. In our focus on calories in/calories out, we've tended not to notice the connection of stress to weight gain and the link between stress hormones like cortisol and fat retention around your waist. The reality of modern life is that it is going to be pressured and hurried. That's simply the reality for most of us. But within that framework, we can make choices that will minimize stress, beat back cortisol and other stress hormones, and help maintain a healthy weight. Therefore, breathe to lose abdominal fat.

Breathing is great for stress reduction. This may seem obvious—after all, you have to breathe no matter what, right? But few of us breathe deeply or consciously. Think about it—when was the last time you took a long, slow, deep breath, and slowly let it out again? Deep breaths of that kind take you out of your immersion in momentary stress, they oxygenate your brain and tissues, and they help to reduce stress hormones. Take breathing breaks throughout the day, or, better yet, pair those breaks with a quiet walk to disassociate from the stress. Just a couple of minutes of walking and a few long, deep breaths, and you will start to see the results in your body.

Flat-Belly Must-Do #6

Adequate sleep is key to a flat belly—tired people can be easily irritated and can make poorer decisions. But sleep also plays into overeating because sleep deprivation can raise levels of ghrelin, a hormone that causes the sensation of hunger. So if you don't get enough sleep (at least 6 hours), you may find yourself unusually hungry the next day—and sooner or later you may break down and snack on the most immediate source of satiation: sugar. Remain sleep deprived over time, and those calories can really add up. Lack of sleep can also alter gut bacteria. The latest research has found strong evidence that not only does our sleep affect our microbiome, but our microbiome also affects our sleep.

What to Do After the First 7 Days

After completing the 7-day flat-belly plan, consider repeating the same week again with some variation by trying new recipes from another season. It is okay to mix and match recipes from spring, summer, fall, and winter. Just make sure to keep all portion sizes where they need to be. Another option is continuing this plan but enjoying some meals outside the flat-belly plan by following these simple rules.

For a flat belly or weight loss, I always recommend using a 90/10 rule with regard to your meals. This just simply means that you follow the plan 90 percent of the week, and the remaining 10 percent can be used for social interactions or personal indulgences. This provides you with two meals outside your meal plan. For instance, on Wednesday, you have a business meeting, and they are serving burgers or a slice of pizza. Please feel free to enjoy them. This will be 1 of your 2 outside meals. The second meal can be that celebratory brunch that you were invited to. Just be sure to be mindful of portion sizes for both food and beverages. You can continue following this rule until you reach your goal weight.

Once you have reached your goal weight, you now should switch gears and begin to focus on weight maintenance. This is where you can switch to an 80/20 rule: follow the plan 80 percent of the week, and the remaining 20 percent can be used for social interactions or personal indulgences.

If you would like to take it a step further for a customized plan, visit *WholeBodyReboot.com*. Whole Body Reboot is a wellness program that encourages eating more nutrient-dense foods, not less. It is an online, interactive, and customized website that tailors a specific meal plan to your needs. It has in-depth tracking tools that help you track your meals, behaviors, mood, and exercise to help you reach your goal. It is also equipped with a mobile app, making it easier for those who are always on the go.

Top Tips When Dining Out

Dine out no more than 1 to 2 times per week for optimal success.

Savor the meal and enjoy it instead of worrying or feeling guilty. By dining out only 1 to 2 times per week and following the meal plans I have provided for you, you will succeed in losing weight. Enjoy the minimal splurges.

Planning ahead makes all the difference. If possible, go online to see the choices available and pick a dish that works for your goals.

If you must eat out more than once or twice a week, you need to be more cautious. Have a snack before going to the restaurant so you are not starving when you get there. You will make better food choices and be less tempted to eat the bread or chips on the table.

Start with a salad or soup. What you'll discover is that, after an appetizer, you may feel fuller. Choose an appetizer as your entrée or bring half of your entrée home.

Ask for sauce and dressing on the side. This may sound obvious, but many people order these as extras on the side and then proceed to pour them all over their meal, using every last drop. It defeats the purpose of getting these on the side in the first place, right? The whole point is that you should use about half of what most restaurants provide. Waiters may tell you things are lightly dressed, but that is rarely the case.

Remember: it's useful to think of eating out as celebratory. I treat it as something exotic and rewarding that I only allow myself once in a while.

CHAPTER 3

The 7-Day Spring Reboot

Spring is often seen as the birth of a new year, with many different species of plants beginning to blossom after the harsh months of winter. It is often associated with rejuvenation, renewal, or having a fresh start, not just with plants, but with people as well. Therefore, we are starting with the spring, showcasing the abundance of green leafy vegetables, berries, and other superfood fruits and vegetables available during this season. The recipes that I include in this season play with different textures of salads, which tend to be light and full of greens, and also soups. I provide broth-based soups that are perfect to keep you warm on a cool spring night. As you can see, there is a quick chart to help you identify the seasonal bounty available at grocery stores and farmers markets.

Table 4: Seasonal Fruits and Vegetables During Spring*

Fruits	Vegetables
Apricots	Artichokes
Apriums	Arugula
California avocados	Asparagus
Cherimoyas	Beets
Cherries	Bok choy
Grapefruits	Broccoli
Guavas	Brussels sprouts
Kumquats	Cabbage
Lemons	Carrots
Limes	Collard greens
Loquats	Dandelion greens
Mandarins	Endives
Oranges	Fava beans
Pomelos	Kale
Rhubarb	Leeks
Strawberries	Mushrooms
	Parsnips
	Pea shoots
	Peas
	Radishes
	Rutabaga

Fruits (continued)	Vegetables (continued)
	Scallions
	Spinach
	Sunchokes
	Swiss chard
	Turnips

* For a downloadable version of this table, visit www.flatbelly365.com/resources

Spring 1,300 Calorie 7-Day Menu

	Monday	Tuesday	Wednesday	Thursday
Breakfast	**2 cups** *Fruity Avocado Smoothie Bowl* (see page 48) TOPPINGS: **4 halves** walnuts **¼ cup** raspberries **¼ cup** pichuberry **1 teaspoon** chia seeds **1 teaspoon** coconut flakes *(see page 25 for other topping options)*	**1 cup** *Chocolate Smoothie Bowl* (see page 49) TOPPINGS: **½ cup** blueberries **¼ cup** strawberries, sliced **¼ cup** oats **1 tablespoon** cacao nibs *(see page 25 for other topping options)*	**2 cups** *Silky Papaya Smoothie* (see page 50) **1** hard-boiled egg	**2 cups** *Fruity Avocado Smoothie Bowl* (see page 48) TOPPINGS: **4 halves** walnuts **¼ cup** raspberries **¼ cup** pichuberry **1 teaspoon** chia seeds **1 teaspoon** coconut flakes *(see page 25 for other topping options)*
Snack	**¾ cup** blueberries or berry of choice *(see Table 3)*	**1 ounce** aged Parmesan cheese **1 medium** pear or fruit of choice *(see Table 3)*	**¾ cup** blueberries or berry of choice *(see Table 3)*	**1 ounce** aged Parmesan cheese **1 medium** pear or fruit of choice *(see Table 3)*
Lunch	**1** *Artichoke-Mint Salad* *(see page 51)* **1 tablespoon** Lemon-Mustard Vinaigrette *(see page 56)* **3 oz.** boneless, skinless chicken breast, baked or grilled or protein of choice *(see Table 2)*	**2 cups** *Beef Bone Soup* *(see page 57)* **1 cup** fermented vegetables *(see page 130)*	**1** *Egg & Avocado Spring Salad* *(see page 53)* **1 tablespoon** Lemon-Mustard Vinaigrette *(see page 56)* **3 oz.** boneless, skinless chicken breast, baked or grilled or protein of choice *(see Table 2)*	**1** *Asparagus-Quinoa Salad (see page 52)* **1 tablespoon** Lemon-Mustard Vinaigrette *(see page 56)* **3 oz.** boneless, skinless chicken breast, baked or grilled or protein of choice *(see Table 2)*
Snack	**1 medium** apple or fruit of choice *(see Table 3)* **12** almonds	**¾ cup** blueberries or berry of choice *(see Table 3)*	**1 medium** apple or fruit of choice *(see Table 3)* **12** almonds	**¾ cup** blueberries or berry of choice *(see Table 3)*
Dinner	**2 cups** *Albondigas Soup* with 2 meatballs *(see page 54)* **1 cup** fermented vegetables *(see page 130)*	**2 cups** *Albondigas Soup* with 2 meatballs *(see page 54)* **1 cup** fermented vegetables *(see page 130)*	**1 serving** *Asparagus-Quinoa Salad* *(see page 52)* **1 tablespoon** Lemon-Mustard Vinaigrette *(see page 56)* **3 oz.** boneless, skinless chicken breast, baked or grilled or protein of choice *(see Table 2)*	**2 cups** *Beef Bone Soup* *(see page 57)* **1 cup** Fermented Vegetables *(see page 130)*

Spring 1,300 Calorie 7-Day Menu (continued)

	Friday	Saturday	Sunday
Breakfast	**2 cups** *Silky Papaya Smoothie* *(see page 50)* **1** hard-boiled egg	**2 cups** *Fruity Avocado Smoothie Bowl* *(see page 48)* TOPPINGS: **4 halves** walnuts **¼ cup** raspberries **¼ cup** pichuberry **1 teaspoon** chia seeds **1 teaspoon** coconut flakes *(see page 25 for other topping options)*	**1 cup** *Chocolate Smoothie Bowl* *(see page 49)* TOPPINGS: **½** cup blueberries **¼** cup strawberries, sliced **¼** cup oats **1** tablespoon cacao nibs *(see page 25 for other topping options)*
Snack	**1** medium apple or fruit of choice *(see Table 3)* **12** almonds	**¾ cup** blueberries or berry of choice *(see Table 4)*	**1** medium apple or fruit of choice *(see Table 3)* **12** almonds
Lunch	**1** *Egg & Avocado Spring Salad* *(see page 53)* **1 tablespoon** Lemon-Mustard Vinaigrette *(see page 56)* **3 oz.** boneless, skinless chicken breast, baked or grilled or protein of choice *(see Table 4)*	**2 cups** *Albondigas Soup* with 2 meatballs *(see page 54)* **1 cup** fermented vegetables *(see page 130)*	**2 cups** *Beef Bone Soup* *(see page 57)* **1 cup** fermented vegetables *(see page 130)*
Snack	**1** medium apple or fruit of choice *(see Table 3)* **12** almonds	**1 ounce** aged Parmesan cheese **1** medium pear or fruit of choice *(see Table 3)*	**¾ cup** blueberries or berry of choice *(see Table 3)*
Dinner	**2 cups** *Albondigas Soup* with 2 meatballs *(see page 54)* **1 cup** fermented vegetables *(see page 130)*	**2 cups** *Beef Bone Soup* *(see page 57)* **1 cup** fermented vegetables *(see page 130)*	**1** *Artichoke-Mint Salad* *(see page 51)* **1 tablespoon** Lemon-Mustard Vinaigrette *(see page 56)* **3 oz.** boneless, skinless chicken breast, baked or grilled or protein of choice *(see Table 4)*

Spring 1,800 Calorie 7-Day Menu

	Monday	Tuesday	Wednesday	Thursday
Breakfast	**2 cups** *Fruity Avocado Smoothie Bowl* (see page 48) TOPPINGS: **4 halves** walnuts **¼ cup** raspberries **¼ cup** pichuberry **1 teaspoon** chia seeds **1 teaspoon** coconut flakes or toppings of choice (see Table 3)	**2 cups** *Chocolate Smoothie Bowl* (see page 49) TOPPINGS: **½ cup** blueberries **¼ cup** strawberries, sliced **¼ cup** oats **1 tablespoon** cacao nibs or toppings of choice (see Table 3)	**2 cups** *Silky Papaya Smoothie* (see page 50) **2 hard-boiled eggs**	**2 cups** *Fruity Avocado Smoothie Bowl* (see page 48) TOPPINGS: **4 halves** walnuts **¼ cup** raspberries **¼ cup** pichuberry **1 teaspoon** chia seeds **1 teaspoon** coconut flakes or toppings of choice (see Table 3)
Snack	**1 cup** blueberries or berry of choice (see Table 4) **8 halves** walnuts	**2 oz** aged Parmesan cheese **1 medium** pear or fruit of choice (see Table 4)	**1 cup** blueberries or berry of choice (see Table 4) **8 halves** walnuts	**2 oz** aged Parmesan cheese **1 medium** pear or fruit of choice (see Table 4)
Lunch	1 Artichoke-Mint Salad (see page 51) **1 tablespoon** Lemon-Mustard Vinaigrette (see page 56) **6 oz** boneless, skinless chicken breast, baked or grilled or protein of choice (see Table 2)	**3 cups** Beef Bone Soup (see page 57) **1 cup** fermented vegetables (see page 130)	1 Egg & Avocado Spring Salad (see page 53) **1 tablespoon** Lemon-Mustard Vinaigrette (see page 56) **6 oz** boneless, skinless chicken breast, baked or grilled or protein of choice (see Table 2)	1 Asparagus-Quinoa Salad (see page 52) **1 tablespoon** Lemon-Mustard Vinaigrette (see page 56) **6 oz** boneless, skinless chicken breast, baked or grilled or protein of choice (see Table 4)
Snack	1 large apple or fruit of choice (see Table 4) **12 almonds**	**1 cup** blueberries or berry of choice (see Table 4) **8 halves** walnuts	1 large apple or fruit of choice (see Table 4) **12 almonds**	**1 cup** blueberries or berry of choice (see Table 4) **8 halves** walnuts
Dinner	**3 cups** *Albondigas Soup with 2 meatballs* (see page 54) **1 cup** fermented vegetables (see page 130)	**3 cups** *Albondigas Soup with 2 meatballs* (see page 54) **1 cup** fermented vegetables (see page 130)	**1 serving** Asparagus-Quinoa Salad (see page 52) **1 tablespoon** Lemon-Mustard Vinaigrette (see page 56) **6 oz.** boneless, skinless chicken breast, baked or grilled or protein of choice (see Table 2)	**3 cups** *Beef Bone Soup* (see page 57) **1 cup** fermented vegetables (see page 130)

Spring 1,800 Calorie 7-Day Menu *(continued)*

	Friday	Saturday	Sunday
Breakfast	**2 cups** *Silky Papaya Smoothie* *(see page 50)* **2** hard-boiled eggs	**2 cups** *Fruity Avocado Smoothie Bowl* *(see page 48)* TOPPINGS: **4 halves** walnuts **¼ cup** raspberries **¼ cup** pichuberry **1 teaspoon** chia seeds **1 teaspoon** coconut flakes or toppings of choice *(see Table 3)*	**2 cups** *Chocolate Smoothie Bowl* *(see page 49)* TOPPINGS: **½ cup** blueberries **¼ cup** strawberries, sliced **¼ cup** oats **1 tablespoon** cacao nibs or toppings of choice *(see Table 3)*
Snack	**1** large apple or fruit of choice *(see Table 4)* **12** almonds	**1 cup** blueberries or berry of choice *(see Table 4)* **8 halves** walnuts	**1** large apple or fruit of choice *(see Table 4)* **12** almonds
Lunch	**1** *Egg & Avocado Spring Salad* *(see page 53)* **1 tablespoon** Lemon-Mustard Vinaigrette *(see page 56)* **6 oz** boneless, skinless chicken breast, baked or grilled or protein of choice *(see Table 2)*	**3 cups** *Albondigas Soup with 2 meatballs* *(see page 54)* **1 cup** fermented vegetables *(see page 130)*	**3 cups** *Beef Bone Soup* *(see page 57)* **1 cup** fermented vegetables *(see page 130)*
Snack	**1** large apple or fruit of choice *(see Table 4)* **12** almonds	**2 ounces** aged Parmesan cheese **1 medium** pear or fruit of choice *(see Table 4)*	**1 cup** blueberries or berry of choice *(see Table 4)* **8 halves** walnuts
Dinner	**3 cups** *Albondigas Soup with 2 meatballs* *(see page 54)* **1 cup** fermented vegetables *(see page 130)*	**3 cups** *Beef Bone Soup* *(see page 57)* **1 cup** fermented vegetables *(see page 130)*	**1** *Artichoke-Mint Salad* *(see page 51)* **1 tablespoon** Lemon-Mustard Vinaigrette *(see page 56)* **6 oz.** boneless, skinless chicken breast, baked or grilled or protein of choice *(see Table 2)*

Fruity Avocado Smoothie Bowl

Servings: 1 ✦ Serving Size: 1 serving

Vegan, Gluten Free

This creamy, fruity bowl is perfect for a spring breakfast. With spinach, pineapple, and avocado, this smoothie bowl delivers an antioxidant punch to get your day started right (see the color photo page 156).

INGREDIENTS

For the base

¾ cup pineapple chunks, frozen

⅓ ripe California avocado, seeded and peeled

¾ cup almond or soy milk, unsweetened

3 cups spinach

1 scoop protein powder* *(whey, soy, pea, or rice)*

The body needs fat to absorb certain phytonutrients and vitamins, such as A, D, K, and E. California avocados, like any other avocados, provide good dietary fats to maximize nutrient absorption.

*Note: To provide 20 grams of protein.

DIRECTIONS

1) Place the pineapple, avocado, almond milk, spinach, and protein powder in a blender. Puree until it reaches a smooth consistency.

2) Pour the smoothie into a medium-sized bowl. Sprinkle with toppings.

Per Serving: Kcal 323, Protein 30g, Carb 32.6g, Fat 12.8g, Sodium 242.2mg, Dietary Fiber 10.5g
Daily Values: Fiber 7%, Vitamin C 142%, Vitamin A 7%, Vitamin D 15%, Potassium 35%, Calcium 54%, Iron 22%

Chocolate Smoothie Bowl

Servings: 2 ✦ Serving Size: 1 cup

Vegan, Gluten Free

It's difficult to say no to the perfect combination of chocolate and banana. With the addition of almond butter, it creates a creamy and smooth texture that will delight your taste buds (see the color photo page 155).

INGREDIENTS for the BASE

1 5-inch banana, frozen

¾ cup almond or soy milk

1 tablespoon almond butter

1 tablespoon cacao powder

1 scoop protein powder* *(whey, soy, pea, or rice)*

*Note: To provide 20 grams of protein.

Cacao polyphenols have been proven to protect against nerve cell injury and inflammation; thus, cacao may play a role in protecting the brain from normal degeneration.

DIRECTIONS

1) Place the banana, almond milk, almond butter, cacao, and protein powder in a blender. Puree until it reaches a smooth consistency.

2) Pour the smoothie into a medium-sized bowl. Sprinkle with toppings (see page 25).

Per Serving: Kcal 206, Protein 17 g, Carb 22 g, Fat 7 g, Sodium 67 mg, Dietary Fiber 3 g,
Daily Values: Fiber 11%, Vitamin C 6%, Vitamin A 6%, Vitamin D 6%, Potassium 12%, Calcium 17%, Iron 5%

Silky Papaya Smoothie

Servings: 1 ✦ Serving Size: 2 cups

Vegan, Gluten Free

Incorporating probiotic and prebiotic foods into your diet is very important to keep you happy and healthy. Kefir offers probiotic strains of bacteria known to be beneficial to our gut system. Papaya also has fiber that makes our stomachs happy.

INGREDIENTS

1 cup low fat plain kefir *(or coconut kefir)*

1 cup papaya, cubed *(or cantaloupe)*

½ cup vanilla soy milk

DIRECTIONS

1) Place kefir, papaya, and vanilla soy milk in a blender. Puree until it reaches the desired consistency.

Papaya contains enzymes called proteolytic enzymes, which are commonly found in the human stomach, that help break down large compounds in the diet. These enzymes, in combination with the fiber content, give papaya the ability to help with digestive system health.

Per Serving: Kcal 275, Protein 19g, Carb 40g, Fat 6g, Sodium 254mg, Dietary Fiber 6.5g
Daily Values: Fiber 24%, Vitamin C 99%, Vitamin A 24%, Vitamin D 35%, Calcium 49%, Iron 11%

Artichoke-Mint Salad

Servings: 1 ✦ Serving Size: 1 serving

Vegan, Gluten Free

The simplicity of this salad is great to showcase a few of the flavors of spring. Artichokes are full of flavor with the added bonus of a burst of nutrition. Mixed in with the cool sensation of mint, this salad is great for any time of day (see the color photo page 151).

INGREDIENTS

2 celery stalks, sliced

1 can (13.75 oz) artichoke hearts, drained

2 tablespoons parsley, chopped

1 tablespoon mint, chopped

1 tablespoon sunflower seeds

Artichokes help protect liver cells. They contain silymarin, which is a flavonoid that supports liver health. Silymarin has been proven to stimulate cell regeneration and fight harmful free radicals.

DIRECTIONS

1) In a medium-sized bowl, add the celery, artichoke hearts, parsley, mint, and sunflower seeds. Toss and mix well.

Per Serving: Kcal 269, Protein 14.0 g, Carb 51 g, Fat 6.0 g, Sodium 302 mg, Dietary Fiber 36 g,
Daily Values: Fiber 128%, Vitamin C 46%, Vitamin A 6%, Vitamin D 0%, Potassium 30%, Calcium 10%, Iron 18%

Asparagus-Quinoa Salad

Servings: 1 ✦ Serving Size: 1 serving

Vegan, Gluten Free

This salad brings out the Latin flavors. Using superfood red quinoa provides plant-based proteins jam packed with all the essential amino acids and anti-oxidants. Combining it with cilantro gives it a Latin twist (see the color photo page 152).

INGREDIENTS

½ cup red quinoa, cooked

8 asparagus spears, peeled and steamed, sliced

2 cups endives, sliced

6 cashews, chopped

2 tablespoons fresh cilantro, chopped

Asparagus is a good source of folate and vitamins A, C, and K. It is also a rich source of glutathione, a detoxifying phytonutrient that helps fight cancer. This superfood also provides prebiotic fiber.

DIRECTIONS

1) In a medium-sized bowl, add the quinoa, asparagus, endives, cashews, and cilantro. Toss well.

2) Add the Lemon-Mustard Vinaigrette *(see page 56)* and dress well.

3) Serve with protein of choice.

Per Serving: Kcal 205, Protein 10 g, Carb 31 g, Fat 6 g, Sodium 37 mg, Dietary Fiber 9 g,
Daily Values: Fiber 32%, Vitamin C 19%, Vitamin A 17%, Vitamin D 0%, Potassium 18% Calcium 8%, Iron 32%

Egg and Avocado Spring Salad

Servings: 1 ✦ Serving Size: 1 serving

Vegetarian, Gluten Free

In California Avocados, the greatest concentration of beneficial carotenoids is in the dark green fruit of the avocado closest to the peel. To get to the nutrient-rich fruit directly under the peel, one should nick and peel the skin from the avocado (see the color photo page 157).

INGREDIENTS

2 radishes, sliced

2 scallions, sliced

1½ cups arugula

2 cups baby romaine lettuce

1 hard-boiled egg, quartered

⅓ ripe California avocado, seeded, peeled, and sliced

Eggs are high in choline, especially the yolk. Choline is an essential nutrient that has been associated with brain health. Recent research shows that eating whole eggs will not raise blood cholesterol.

DIRECTIONS

1) In a medium bowl, add the radishes, scallions, arugula, and romaine lettuce. Toss and mix well.

2) Top with the egg and sliced avocado.

Per Serving: Kcal 182, Protein 10 g, Carb 10 g, Fat 12 g, Sodium 87 mg, Dietary Fiber 5g,
Daily Values: Fiber 20%, Vitamin C 46%, Vitamin A 31%, Vitamin D 6%, Potassium 10%, Calcium 12%, Iron 18%

Chicken Albondigas Soup

Servings: 4 ✦ Serving Size: 2 cups

Gluten Free

In Latin culture, *albondigas* means meatballs. Typically, albondigas are something that your grandmother makes. This easy recipe brings together flavors from Latin America and the United States from cilantro to California Avocado (see the color photo page 154).

INGREDIENTS for the MEATBALLS

1 pound ground chicken

¾ cup cooked brown rice *(¼ cup dry)*

¼ cup red onion, diced

¼ cup green bell pepper, diced

½ teaspoon sea salt

¼ teaspoon black pepper

A one-third serving size of heart-healthy California Avocados contribute nearly twenty vitamins, minerals, and phytonutrients, including 11 percent of the Daily Value (DV) fiber, 10 percent DV folate, and 6 percent DV vitamin E and potassium.

INGREDIENTS for the SOUP

8 cups low sodium chicken broth

½ green bell pepper, sliced

½ red onion, sliced

3 celery stalks, sliced

1 cup carrots, sliced

½ cup fresh cilantro, chopped

1 teaspoon sea salt

½ teaspoon black pepper

1⅓ ripe California avocado, sliced

DIRECTIONS

For the meatballs

1) In a medium bowl, add the ground chicken, rice, onion, diced bell pepper, salt, and black pepper. Mix thoroughly and shape into eight 2¼-oz meatballs with a 2-inch diameter.

2) In a medium-sized pot, pour in the chicken broth and bring to a boil on medium-high heat. Add the chicken and cook for 10 minutes.

3) Add the bell pepper, onion, celery, carrots, cilantro, salt, and black pepper. Cook for 5 minutes or until the vegetables are tender.

4) Serve soup with avocado on top.

Note: In Latin culture, we squeeze lime juice on everything to bring out the flavors. This soup goes well with a squeeze or two. Give it a try.

Per Serving: Kcal 390, Protein 32 g, Carb 26 g, Fat 19 g, Sodium 490 mg, Dietary Fiber 6 g,
Daily Values: Fiber 22%, Vitamin C 38%, Vitamin A 30%, Vitamin D 0%, Potassium 33%, Calcium 6%, Iron 16%

Lemon-Mustard Vinaigrette

Servings: 10 ✦ Serving Size: 1 tablespoon

Vegan, Gluten Free

This zesty and simple vinaigrette can be used on a host of different salads or protein choices. The best part is that a little goes a long way.

INGREDIENTS

½ cup lemon juice

1 teaspoon yellow mustard

¼ teaspoon black pepper

½ teaspoon dried basil

½ teaspoon sea salt

1 tablespoon olive oil

Olive oil is rich in monounsaturated fat or MUFAs, which have been shown to target body fat where it is the hardest to lose: the belly.

DIRECTIONS

1) Put all the ingredients in a small bowl. Whisk together and let sit for 10 minutes. Stir before each use.

Per Serving: Kcal 15, Protein 0g, Carb 1.1g, Fat 1.4g, Sodium 94mg, Dietary Fiber 0g,
Daily Values: Fiber 0%, Vitamin C 9%, Vitamin A 0%, Vitamin D 0%, Potassium 0%, Calcium 0%, Iron 0%

Beef Bone Soup

Servings: 6 ✦ Serving Size: 2 cups

Gluten Free

During the spring, there are many vegetables that are just coming into season. This soup is truly a seasonal feast with a variety of vegetables, perfectly blended with beef shank to make it a hearty soup (see the color photo page 153).

INGREDIENTS

8 cups beef broth

2 pounds beef shank, bone in, cut into 1-inch cubes

1 pound sirloin steak, cut into 1-inch cubes

8 cups Swiss chard, sliced

3 bay leaves

1 medium red onion, cut in quarters

1 cup carrots, cut into ½-inch slice

3 celery stalks, sliced

3 ounces white button mushrooms, sliced

1 cup peas

1½ teaspoons sea salt

Cooking with beef bone not only adds more flavor, but it also enriches the soup with minerals and collagen, both of which support the immune system. Studies show that gelatin is beneficial to restoring gut strength by promoting the growth of probiotics.

DIRECTIONS

1) In a large pot on medium high heat, pour in the beef broth and bring to a boil. Then add the beef and bones, Swiss chard, and bay leaves. Cook for 10 minutes and lower to medium heat.

2) Add the onions, carrots, celery, mushrooms, peas, and salt. Cover and cook for 20 minutes.

If using frozen peas, add at the very end.

Per Serving: Kcal 399, Protein 45g, Carb 27g, Fat 12g, Sodium 1461mg, Dietary Fiber 6g,
Daily Values: Fiber 20%, Vitamin C 34%, Vitamin A 53%, Vitamin D .5%, Potassium 325%, Calcium 7%, Iron 40%

Shiitake Bean Sprout Soup

Servings: 4 ✦ Serving Size: 3 cups

Vegan, Gluten Free

"Pho" is traditionally a Vietnamese noodle soup. Here, I have taken that same flavor concept and added my own twist by using seasonal California vegetables.

INGREDIENTS

½ teaspoon anise seeds

2 cinnamon sticks

1 teaspoon cloves

8 cups vegetable stock

1 medium white onion, chopped

2 inch ginger slice, cut in half

8 ounces shiitake mushrooms, sliced,
    and stems set aside

3 tablespoons soy sauce

2 tablespoons rice vinegar

3 scallions, sliced

4 bok choy, sliced in half

2 cups edamame

9 ounces bean sprouts

Shiitake mushrooms provide B-complex vitamins that help boost your metabolism. If mushrooms are exposed to sunlight as they grow, they become a source of vitamin D in your diet.

DIRECTIONS

1) In a medium-sized pan on medium-high heat, add the anise seeds, cinnamon, and cloves. Roast for 1 minute.

2) Add the vegetable stock, onion, garlic, ginger, and mushroom stems. Bring to a boil and then lower the temperature to low. Simmer for 20 minutes.

3) Strain and return the liquid to the pot. Add the mushroom caps, soy sauce, rice vinegar, and scallions. Simmer for 10 minutes.

4) Add the bok choy and simmer for another 8 minutes.

5) Add the edamame and bean sprouts. Simmer for another 5 minutes.

6) Serve with protein of choice.

Per Serving: Kcal 270, Protein 27 g, Carb 39 g, Fat 7 g, Sodium 2425 mg, Dietary Fiber 16.0 g,
Daily Values: Fiber 58%, Vitamin C 439%, Vitamin A 209%, Vitamin D 1%, Potassium 61%, Calcium 76%, Iron 58%

Spring Shopping List

This shopping list contains only the ingredients that are needed for the recipes included in the 7-day menu plans. If you choose to replace a recipe with another one, please be sure to look at the recipe before shopping and buy the proper ingredients. For a downloadable version of this shopping list, visit *www.flatbelly365.com/resources*.

Produce

❑ 1 pound raspberries

❑ 2 pounds blueberries*

❑ 1 pound strawberries

❑ 5 medium apples

❑ 2 small bananas*

❑ 4 California avocados*

❑ 1 whole papaya

❑ 2 lemons

❑ 8 celery stalks*

❑ 1 green bell pepper*

❑ 1 bunch (1 pound) asparagus spears

❑ 1 head endive

❑ 6 carrots*

❑ 2 medium red onions*

❑ 1 (8 oz) package white button mushrooms*

❑ 2 pounds Swiss chard*

❑ 1 bunch scallions

❑ 1 (9 oz) bag spinach

❑ 1 bunch radishes

❑ 1 (5 oz) bag arugula

❑ 1 (5 oz) bag baby romaine lettuce

❑ 1 bunch fresh cilantro

❑ 1 bunch parsley

❑ 1 bunch mint

Dairy and Eggs

❑ 1 quart container almond or soy milk, unsweetened

❑ 1 (16 oz) container plain, low fat kefir

❑ 1 (8 oz) package aged Parmesan cheese

❑ Half dozen eggs

Pantry

❑ 1 (2 lb) bag brown rice

❑ 1 (12 oz) box red quinoa

❑ 1 (18 oz) container dry oats

❑ 1 (8 oz) bottle yellow mustard or mustard of choice

❑ 1 (8 oz) bag chia seeds

❑ 1 (8 oz) bag sunflower seeds

❑ 2 (32 fl. oz) containers low sodium chicken stock*

❑ 2 (32 fl. oz) containers low sodium beef stock*

❑ 1 (16 oz) bag cashews

❑ 1 (16 oz) bag almonds

❑ 1 (16 oz) bag chopped walnuts

❑ 1 (16 oz) container almond butter

❑ 1 (8 oz) bag cacao powder

❑ 3 cans (13.75 oz) artichoke hearts

❑ Olive oil

❑ Canola oil

Frozen

❑ 1 (16 oz) bag pineapple chunks, frozen

❑ 1 bag (1 lb) frozen peas

Meats or Vegetarian Meats

❑ 1 pound ground chicken*

❑ 2 pounds bone-in beef shank*

❑ 2 pounds boneless, skinless chicken breast or lean protein of choice*

❑ Other choices: White fish, canned tuna, salmon, shrimp, pork loin, sirloin steak, tofu, tempeh, and seitan

Herbs and Spices

❑ Sea salt

❑ Black pepper

❑ Dried basil

Other

❑ Protein powder* *(whey, soy, pea, or rice)*

* Denotes items that need to be doubled for 1,800 calorie menu

CHAPTER 4

The 7-Day Summer Reboot

Typically known for having the longest, hottest days, summer is the perfect season to participate in outdoor activities such as hiking, camping, biking, running, hitting the road on a road trip, or simply planning a vacation to a tropical location. Whatever the case may be, it is also the perfect time to properly fuel yourself with seasonal fruits and vegetables. Here I begin to play with the temperature of some of the recipes by incorporating cold soups, or gazpachos, to help quench your hunger and your thirst. I also switch gears with the salads by making them into mixed grain bowls, incorporating herbs and spices to add flavor and nutrition. I also introduce new smoothies that include mixed berries and other tropical fruits. This quick chart helps you identify the seasonal bounty available at grocery stores and farmers markets.

Table 5: Seasonal Fruits and Vegetables During Summer*

Fruits	Vegetables
Apricots	Arugula
Aprium	Beets
California avocados	Bok Choy
Blackberries	Broccoli
Blueberries	Cabbage
Boysenberries	Carrots
Cactus pears	Celery
Cherries	Chicory
Figs	Collard greens
Grapes	Corn
Lemons	Cucumbers
Loquats	Eggplant
Melons	Endives
Mulberries	Fava beans
Nectarines	Fennel
Oranges	Green beans
Peaches	Kale
Plums	Leeks
Pluots	Mushrooms
Raspberries	Okra
Rhubarb	Peppers (sweet and chili)

Fruits *(continued)*	Vegetables *(continued)*
Strawberries	Potatoes
Tayberries	Purslane
Watermelon	Radishes
	Shallots
	Spinach
	Sprouts
	Summer squash
	Swiss chard
	Tomatoes
	Tomatillos

*For a downloadable version of this table, visit www.flatbelly365.com/resources

Summer 1,300 Calorie 7-Day Menu

	Monday	Tuesday	Wednesday	Thursday
Breakfast	1½ **cups** *Berry Mango Smoothie* *(see page 72)*	½ **cup** Greek yogurt, plain, 2% fat 1 **cup** raspberries or berry of choice *(see Table 4)*	2 **cups** *Peach Papaya Smoothie* *(see page 71)*	1½ **cups** *Berry Mango Smoothie* *(see page 72)*
Snack	2 **cups** watermelon or fruit of choice *(see Table 5)* 1 **tablespoon** sunflower seeds	1 **cup** whole strawberries or berry of choice *(see Table 5)* 12 almonds	1 **cup** whole strawberries or berry of choice *(see Table 5)* 12 almonds	2 **cups** watermelon or fruit of choice *(see Table 5)* 1 **tablespoon** sunflower seeds
Lunch	1½ **cups** *Sweet Corn Gazpacho* *(see page 74)* 3 **oz** boneless, skinless chicken breast, baked or grilled or protein of choice *(see Table 2)*	1 *Fig Jicama Salad* *(see page 75)* 2 **tablespoons** Roasted Strawberry Vinaigrette *(see page 83)* 3 **oz** boneless, skinless chicken breast, baked or grilled or protein of choice *(see Table 2)*	½ **cup** *Walnut Pesto Quinoa Bowl* *(see page 80)* 3.5 **cups** mixed greens salad with lemon juice and salt	1 *Fig Jicama Salad* *(see page 75)* 2 **tablespoons** Roasted Strawberry Vinaigrette *(see page 83)* 3 **oz** boneless, skinless chicken breast, baked or grilled or protein of choice *(see Table 2)*
Snack	1 medium nectarine or fruit of choice *(see Table 5)* 15 pistachios	1 **cup** Fermented Vegetables *(see page 130)* 1 **oz** aged Parmesan cheese	1 medium nectarine or fruit of choice *(see Table 5)* 15 pistachios	1 **cup** Fermented Vegetables *(see page 130)* 1 **oz** aged Parmesan cheese
Dinner	1 *Fig Jicama Salad* *(see page 75)* 2 **tablespoons** Roasted Strawberry Vinaigrette *(see page 83)* 3 **oz** boneless, skinless chicken breast, baked or grilled or protein of choice *(see Table 2)*	½ **cup** *Walnut Pesto Quinoa Bowl* *(see page 80)* 3.5 **cups** mixed greens salad with lemon juice and salt	1½ **cups** *Sweet Corn Gazpacho* *(see page 74)* 3 **oz** boneless, skinless chicken breast, baked or grilled or protein of choice *(see Table 2)*	½ **cup** *Walnut Pesto Quinoa Bowl* *(see page 80)* 3.5 **cups** mixed greens salad with lemon juice and salt

Summer 1,300 Calorie 7-Day Menu *(continued)*

	Friday	Saturday	Sunday
Breakfast	½ cup Greek yogurt, plain, 2% fat 1 cup raspberries or berry of choice *(see Table 4)*	2 cups Peach Papaya Smoothie *(see page 71)*	1½ cups Berry Mango Smoothie *(see page 72)*
Snack	1 cup whole strawberries or berry of choice *(see Table 5)* 12 almonds	2 cups watermelon or fruit of choice *(see Table 5)* 1 tablespoon sunflower seeds	1 cup whole strawberries or berry of choice *(see Table 5)* 12 almonds
Lunch	1 *Avocado Mango Salad* *(see page 76)* 1 tablespoon Lemon-Mustard Vinaigrette *(see page 56)* 3 oz boneless, skinless chicken breast, baked or grilled or protein of choice *(see Table 2)*	1½ cups *Sweet Corn Gazpacho* *(see page 74)* 3 oz boneless, skinless chicken breast, baked or grilled or protein of choice *(see Table 2)*	1 *Avocado Mango Salad* *(see page 76)* 1 tablespoon Lemon-Mustard Vinaigrette *(see page 56)* 3 oz boneless, skinless chicken breast, baked or grilled or protein of choice *(see Table 2)*
Snack	1 medium nectarine or fruit of choice *(see Table 5)* 15 pistachios	1 medium nectarine or fruit of choice *(see Table 5)* 15 pistachios	1 cup Fermented Vegetables *(see page 130)* 1 oz aged Parmesan cheese
Dinner	1½ cups *Sweet Corn Gazpacho* *(see page 74)* 3 oz boneless, skinless chicken breast, baked or grilled or protein of choice *(see Table 2)*	1 *Avocado Mango Salad* *(see page 76)* 1 tablespoon Lemon-Mustard Vinaigrette *(see page 56)* 3 oz boneless, skinless chicken breast, baked or grilled or protein of choice *(see Table 2)*	½ cup *Walnut Pesto Quinoa Bowl* *(see page 80)* 3½ cups mixed greens salad with lemon juice and salt

Summer 1,800 Calorie 7-Day Menu

	Monday	Tuesday	Wednesday	Thursday
Breakfast	1½ **cups** *Berry Mango Smoothie* (see page 72)	1 **cup** Greek yogurt, plain, 2% fat 1 **cup** raspberries or berry of choice (see Table 5)	2 **cups** *Peach Papaya Smoothie* (see page 71)	1½ cups *Berry Mango Smoothie* (see page 72)
Snack	2 **cups** watermelon or fruit of choice (see Table 5) 3 **tablespoons** sunflower seeds	1 **cup** whole strawberries or berry of choice (see Table 5) 18 almonds	1 **cup** whole strawberries or berry of choice (see Table 5) 18 almonds	2 **cups** watermelon or fruit of choice (see Table 5) 3 **tablespoons** sunflower seeds
Lunch	3 **cups** *California Avocado Gazpacho* (see page 73) 6 **oz.** boneless, skinless chicken breast, baked or grilled or protein of choice (see Table 2)	1 *Fig Jicama Salad* (see page 75) 2 **tablespoons** Roasted Strawberry Vinaigrette (see page 83) 6 **oz.** boneless, skinless chicken breast, baked or grilled or protein of choice (see Table 2)	½ **cup** *Walnut Pesto Quinoa Bowl* (see page 80) 3 **oz.** boneless, skinless chicken breast, baked or grilled or protein of choice (see Table 2) 3½ **cups** mixed greens salad with lemon juice and salt	1 *Fig Jicama Salad* (see page 75) 2 **tablespoons** Roasted Strawberry Vinaigrette (see page 83) 6 **oz.** boneless, skinless chicken breast, baked or grilled or protein of choice (see Table 2)
Snack	1 medium nectarine or fruit of choice (see Table 5) 30 pistachios	1 **cup** Fermented Vegetables (see page 130) 2 **ounces** aged Parmesan cheese	1 medium nectarine or fruit of choice (see Table 5) 30 pistachios	1 **cup** Fermented Vegetables (see page 130) 2 **oz.** aged Parmesan cheese
Dinner	1 *Fig Jicama Salad* (see page 75) 2 **tablespoons** Roasted Strawberry Vinaigrette (see page 83) 3 **oz.** boneless, skinless chicken breast, baked or grilled or protein of choice (see Table 2) 3½ **cups** mixed greens salad with lemon juice and salt	½ **cup** *Walnut Pesto Quinoa Bowl* (see page 80) 3 **oz.** boneless, skinless chicken breast, baked or grilled or protein of choice (see Table 3) 3½ **cups** mixed greens salad with lemon juice and salt	3 **cups** *California Avocado Gazpacho* (see page 73) 6 **oz.** boneless, skinless chicken breast, baked or grilled or protein of choice (see Table 2)	½ **cup** *Walnut Pesto Quinoa Bowl* (see page 80) 3 **oz.** boneless, skinless chicken breast, baked or grilled or protein of choice (see Table 2) 3½ **cups** mixed greens salad with lemon juice and salt

Summer 1,800 Calorie 7-Day Menu *(continued)*

	Friday	Saturday	Sunday
Breakfast	**1 cup** Greek yogurt, plain, 2% fat 1 cup raspberries or berry of choice *(see Table 5)*	**2 cups** *Peach Papaya Smoothie* *(see page 71)*	**1½ cups** *Berry Mango Smoothie* *(see page 72)*
Snack	**1 cup** whole strawberries or berry of choice *(see Table 5)* **18** almonds	**2 cups** watermelon or fruit of choice *(see Table 5)* **3 tablespoons** sunflower seeds	**1 cup** whole strawberries or berry of choice *(see Table 5)* **18** almonds
Lunch	**1** *Avocado Mango Salad* *(see page 76)* **1 tablespoon** Lemon-Mustard Vinaigrette *(see page 56)* **6 oz.** boneless, skinless chicken breast, baked or grilled or protein of choice *(see Table 2)*	**3 cups** *Sweet Corn Gazpacho* *(see page 74)* **6 oz.** boneless, skinless chicken breast, baked or grilled or protein of choice *(see Table 2)*	**1** *Avocado Mango Salad* *(see page 76)* **1 tablespoon** Lemon-Mustard Vinaigrette *(see page 56)* **6 oz.** boneless, skinless chicken breast, baked or grilled or protein of choice *(see Table 2)*
Snack	**1** medium nectarine or fruit of choice *(see Table 5)* **30** pistachios	**1** medium nectarine or fruit of choice *(see Table 5)* **30** pistachios	**1 cup** Fermented Vegetables *(see page 130)* **2 oz.** aged Parmesan cheese
Dinner	**3 cups** *Sweet Corn Gazpacho* *(see page 74)* **6 oz.** boneless, skinless chicken breast, baked or grilled or protein of choice *(see Table 2)*	**1** *Avocado Mango Salad* *(see page 76)* **1 tablespoon** Lemon-Mustard Vinaigrette *(see page 56)* **6 oz.** boneless, skinless chicken breast, baked or grilled or protein of choice *(see Table 2)*	**½ cup** *Walnut Pesto Quinoa Bowl* *(see page 80)* **3 oz.** boneless, skinless chicken breast, baked or grilled or protein of choice *(see Table 2)* **3½ cups** mixed greens salad with lemon juice and salt

Watermelon Strawberry Smoothie

Servings: 1 ✦ Serving Size: 1 serving

Vegan, Gluten Free

When you think of watermelon, you think of eating it by itself on a hot summer day with its natural sweetness dancing on your tongue. Here I go one step further by combining it with strawberries and cucumber to showcase the freshness of this smoothie (see the color photo page 164).

INGREDIENTS

1¼ cups watermelon

1 cup strawberries

1 cup cucumber, peeled and sliced

¼ cup celery, sliced

1 tablespoon chia seeds

1 tablespoon lemon juice

1 scoop protein powder* *(whey, soy, or pea)*

Note: To provide 20 grams of protein.

Watermelon is 92 percent water and a good source of fiber. The combination of water and fiber means that you are eating a good volume of food without a lot of calories. This helps you feel not just hydrated, but also full.

DIRECTIONS

1) Place all the ingredients in a blender and puree until the smoothie reaches the desired consistency.

Per Serving: Kcal 306, Protein 29g, Carb 38 g, Fat 7 g, Sodium 76 mg, Dietary Fiber 10 g,
Daily Values: Fiber 34%, Vitamin C 122%, Vitamin A 7%, Vitamin D 0%, Potassium 18%, Calcium 21%, Iron 13%

Peach Papaya Smoothie

Servings: 1 ✦ Serving Size: 1 serving

Vegan, Gluten Free

Nothing screams summer like the flavor of a peach. Peach is not only distinct in its flavor, but also in its versatility. People often use peaches in salads, desserts, and, sometimes, alcohol. Here, I keep it simple with a delicious smoothie to start off your morning.

INGREDIENTS

1 whole peach, core removed

1 cup papaya, diced

½ cup carrots, sliced

1 cup yellow zucchini, sliced

1 tablespoon chia seeds

1 tablespoon lemon juice

1 cup water

1 scoop protein powder* *(whey, soy, pea, or rice)*

Note: To provide 20 grams of protein.

Chia seeds are high in omega-3 and omega-6 fatty acids, which help the body stabilize blood sugar and slow down carbohydrate metabolism.

DIRECTIONS

1) Place all the ingredients in a blender and puree until the smoothie reaches the desired consistency.

Per Serving: Kcal 346, Protein 30g, Carb 47 g, Fat 8 g, Sodium 112 mg, Dietary Fiber 13.1 g,
Daily Values: Fiber 45%, Vitamin C 139%, Vitamin A 68%, Vitamin D 0%, Potassium 26%, Calcium 22%, Iron 12%

Berry Mango Smoothie

Servings: 1 ✦ Serving Size: 1 serving

Vegan, Gluten Free

Adding the tropical flavors of mango to the seasonal notes of strawberries is the perfect way to enjoy this season's best smoothie.

INGREDIENTS

¾ cup mango

1 cup strawberries

1 cup cucumber

1 cup yellow zucchini

1 tablespoon chia seeds

2 mint leaves

1 tablespoon lemon juice

1 cup water

1 scoop protein powder* *(whey, soy, or pea)*

Note: To provide 20 grams of protein.

Clinical research suggests that eating strawberries is good for the whole body. It promotes heart health and diabetes management, supports brain health, and reduces the risk of some cancers.

DIRECTIONS

1) Place all the ingredients in a blender and puree until the smoothie reaches the desired consistency.

Per Serving: Kcal 357, Protein 30g, Carb 50 g, Fat 8 g, Sodium 64 mg, Dietary Fiber 12 g,
Daily Values: Fiber 43%, Vitamin C 189%, Vitamin A 11%, Vitamin D 0%, Potassium 24%, Calcium 22%, Iron 14%

California Avocado Gazpacho

Servings: 4 ✦ Serving Size: 1½ cups

Vegan, Gluten Free

California avocados are a delicious, nutritious superfruit that are locally and responsibly grown on nearly 4,000 family farms throughout central and southern California. Summer is the peak season for this superfood that adds a rich, creamy flavor to this refreshing gazpacho (see the color photo page 159).

INGREDIENTS

1 medium cucumber, peeled and chopped

½ medium red onion, chopped

1 pound yellow cherry tomatoes

1 ripe California avocado, seeded and peeled

1 green bell pepper, chopped

¼ cup parsley, chopped

½ cup vegetable stock

¼ cup white wine vinegar

1 teaspoon garlic, minced

1 tablespoon aji amarillo or other chili paste

1 tablespoon lime juice

1½ teaspoons sea salt

California avocados contribute good fats, such as monounsaturated fats, to your diet. Good fats do not raise LDL "bad" cholesterol levels, and monounsaturated fats are known to be anti-inflammatory.

DIRECTIONS

1) Place all the ingredients in a blender. Puree until they reach the desired consistency.

2) Refrigerate for 1 hour before serving to allow the flavors to marinate.

Per Serving: Kcal 101, Protein 3 g, Carb 12 g, Fat 6 g, Sodium 792 mg, Dietary Fiber 4g,
Daily Values: Fiber 15%, Vitamin C 59%, Vitamin A 5%, Vitamin D 0%, Potassium 14%, Calcium 3%, Iron 8%

Sweet Corn Gazpacho

Servings: 4 ✦ Serving Size: 1½ cups

Vegan, Gluten Free

Who says corn only belongs on the grill? This tasty gazpacho brings out the sweetness of the corn while also giving you a refreshing burst of flavor (see the color photo page 161).

INGREDIENTS

3 ears of corn, cooked and cooled

12 ounces yellow cherry tomatoes

1 yellow bell pepper, chopped

½ medium red onion, chopped

2 celery stalks, sliced

¾ cup vegetable broth

¼ cup white wine vinegar

1 tablespoon chili powder

3 tablespoons lime juice

1 teaspoon garlic, minced

1½ teaspoons sea salt

¼ teaspoon black pepper

Foods such as red onions, bell peppers, and garlic are good prebiotic sources. Prebiotics help the good bacteria in your gut multiply.

DIRECTIONS

1) Place all the ingredients in a blender. Puree until they reach the desired consistency.

2) Refrigerate for 1 hour before serving to let the flavors marinate.

Per Serving: Kcal 110, Protein 4 g, Carb 23 g, Fat 2 g, Sodium 936 mg, Dietary Fiber 4 g,
Daily Values: Fiber 13%, Vitamin C 114%, Vitamin A 5%, Vitamin D 0%, Potassium 14%, Calcium 3%, Iron 8%

Fig Jicama Salad

Servings: 1 ✦ Serving Size: 1 serving

Vegan, Gluten Free

Figs are at peak perfection during the summer months, so I wanted to keep their gorgeous flavor alive. With jicama and garbanzo beans, this salad explodes with Mediterranean flavors (see the color photo page 160).

INGREDIENTS

2 medium-sized figs, quartered

1 cup jicama, peeled and cut into small cubes

¼ cup red onion, sliced thin

¼ cup cucumber, peeled and quartered

½ cup garbanzo beans

Lemon-Mustard Vinaigrette *(see page 56)*

Figs are high in both soluble and insoluble fiber. Soluble fiber slows digestion, making you feel more satisfied. Insoluble fiber promotes regularity, which helps cleanse the large intestine and eliminate waste.

DIRECTIONS

1) In a medium bowl, place the figs, jicama, onion, cucumber, and garbanzo beans. Toss and mix well.

2) Add the Lemon-Mustard Vinaigrette. Toss and dress well.

3) Serve with protein of choice.

Per Serving: Kcal 216, Protein 8 g, Carb 43 g, Fat 3 g, Sodium 343.0 mg, Dietary Fiber 14 g,
Daily Values: Fiber 50%, Vitamin C 33%, Vitamin A .5%, Vitamin D 0%, Potassium 12%, Calcium 8%, Iron 15%

Avocado Mango Salad

Servings: 1 ✦ Serving Size: 1 serving

Vegan, Gluten Free

This refreshing salad combines the bright, sweet flavor of mango with the delicious, creamy texture of avocado. A one-third serving of avocado contains 10 percent of Daily Values of fiber. Moreover, diets rich in heathy foods containing fiber, such as some fruits and vegetables, may reduce the risk of heart disease, obesity, and type 2 diabetes (see the color photo page 158).

INGREDIENTS

⅓ ripe California avocado, peeled, seeded, and diced

½ cup mango, diced

½ cup fennel, sliced thin

1 medium tomato, cut into ⅛-inch slices

¼ cup parsley, chopped

4 halves of walnuts

4 cups arugula

Roasted Strawberry Vinaigrette *(see page 83)*

Mangos are bursting with antioxidants and over twenty different vitamins and minerals. In just a one cup serving, mangos provide you with 100 percent of your daily requirement of vitamin C.

DIRECTIONS

1) In a medium bowl, place the avocado, mango, fennel, tomato, parsley, walnuts, and arugula. Toss and mix well.

2) Add the Roasted Strawberry Vinaigrette. Toss and dress well.

3) Serve with protein of choice.

Per Serving: Kcal 242, Protein 7 g, Carb 29 g, Fat 14 g, Sodium 64 mg, Dietary Fiber 10 g,
Daily Values: Fiber 34%, Vitamin C 98%, Vitamin A 31%, Vitamin D 0%, Potassium 27%, Calcium 16%, Iron 19%

Tomato Beet Salad

Servings: 1 ✦ Serving Size: 1 serving

Vegan, Gluten Free

Tomatoes and beets are a great combination, as both have a natural sweetness and carry earthy and savory notes that are perfect for any dish (see the color photo page 162).

INGREDIENTS

1 medium-sized tomato, cut into ⅛-inch slices

½ cup red beets, cooked

½ cup golden beets, cooked

¼ cup red onion, sliced thin

6 almonds, chopped

3 basil leaves, sliced

Lemon-Mustard Vinaigrette *(see page 56)*

Beets are rich in betaine, as well as folate; both work synergistically to help reduce the risk of artery damage and heart disease.

DIRECTIONS

1) In a medium bowl, place the tomato, beets, onion, almonds, and basil. Toss and mix well.

2) Add the Lemon-Mustard Vinaigrette. Toss and dress well.

3) Serve with protein of choice.

Per Serving: Kcal 155, Protein 6 g, Carb 27 g, Fat 4 g, Sodium 139 mg, Dietary Fiber 6 g,
Daily Values: Fiber 23%, Vitamin C 29%, Vitamin A 7%, Vitamin D 0%, Potassium 20%, Calcium 7%, Iron 12%

Grilled Fruit and Vegetable Salad

Servings: 4 ✦ Serving Size: 3 cups

Vegan, Gluten Free

This recipe takes salad to a whole new level. Grilling fruits and vegetables brings out their natural sweetness, adding a different dimension of flavor and texture.

INGREDIENTS

1 large red onion, sliced

4 large heirloom tomatoes, cut into quarters

2 ripe California avocados, cut into quarters and peeled

2 mangos, peeled and cut into wedges

Canola oil spray

1 teaspoon sea salt

4 cups arugula

Cilantro-Lime Dressing *(see page 82)*

Adding different colored fruits and vegetables to your diet allows you to capitalize on the full range of benefits—vitamins, minerals, phytonutrients, and antioxidants—found in each food.

DIRECTIONS

1) Preheat your grill to 400°F.

2) Place all the vegetables and fruits in a large bowl. Spray with canola oil spray, making sure to coat them all evenly. Sprinkle with salt.

3) Spray the grill with oil and place the vegetables and fruits on the grill. Cook for 2 to 3 minutes or until grill marks begin to show. Turn them over and cook for another 2 to 3 minutes. For fruits and vegetables such as mango, avocado, and tomato, you may need to turn it on a third side, depending on your preference.

4) In a large bowl, place the arugula at the bottom. Then collect the grilled vegetables and fruits in the bowl. The heat will wilt the arugula a bit.

5) Drizzle the dressing on top.

Nutrition facts, without dressing
Per Serving: Kcal 239, Protein 4g, Carb 30g, Fat 14g, Sodium 596mg, Dietary Fiber 9g,
Daily Values: Fiber 31%, Vitamin C 80%, Vitamin A 15%, Vitamin D 0%, Potassium 21%, Calcium 6%, Iron 8%

Walnut Pesto Quinoa Bowl

Servings: 4 ◆ Serving Size: ½ cup quinoa and 1 tablespoon pesto

Vegetarian, Gluten Free

This is one of my favorite dishes because it combines the nutritional power of quinoa with the versatile flavors of basil and spinach. What's even better? This dish can be eaten for breakfast, lunch, or dinner (see the color photo page 163).

INGREDIENTS for the QUINOA

1 cup red quinoa, raw

1¾ cups vegetable stock

1 cup red bell pepper, diced small

½ teaspoon sea salt

1 poached egg, for garnish

Quinoa has a low glycemic index of 35. To lose belly fat, quinoa is a great carbohydrate source because it affects blood sugar at a slow rate.

INGREDIENTS for the PESTO

1 tablespoon olive oil

¼ cup red onion, diced

3 cups spinach

2–3 leaves basil

1 tablespoon lemon juice

¼ cup vegetable stock

¼ cup walnuts, chopped

½ teaspoon sea salt

¼ teaspoon black pepper

DIRECTIONS

1) For quinoa: In a small saucepan, place the quinoa, vegetable stock, red bell pepper, and sea salt. Bring it up to a boil, then simmer. Cook for 15 minutes or until the quinoa is cooked. Set aside and cool.

2) For pesto: In a small sauté pan on medium-high heat, place the olive oil and heat for 1 minute. Add the onion and cook for 3 to 5 minutes or until the onion becomes translucent. Remove from the pan and place in a blender.

3) Add the spinach, basil, lemon juice, vegetable stock, walnuts, salt, and black pepper to the blender. Puree until the mixture reaches a smooth, thick consistency.

4) Place the quinoa mixture in a medium-sized bowl. Add 4 tablespoons of the pesto to the bowl and mix thoroughly. Place a poached egg on top.

5) Refrigerate remaining pesto for later use. It keeps for up to 5 days.

Note: For every ½ cup of quinoa, add 1 tablespoon of pesto.

For quinoa and 1 tablespoon pesto
Per Serving: Kcal 215, Protein 9 g, Carb 31 g, Fat 7 g, Sodium 578 mg, Dietary Fiber 4 g,
Daily Values: Fiber 15%, Vitamin C 56%, Vitamin A 13%, Vitamin D 1%, Potassium 9%, Calcium 3%, Iron 15%

For pesto only
Servings: 12 • Serving Size: 1 tablespoon
Per Serving: Kcal 29, Protein 1g, Carb 1g, Fat 3g, Sodium 80mg, Dietary Fiber 0g,
Daily Values: Fiber 1%, Vitamin C 3%, Vitamin A 4%, Vitamin D 0%, Potassium 1%, Calcium 1%, Iron 2%

Cilantro-Lime Dressing

Servings: 10 ✦ Serving Size: 2 tablespoons

Vegan, Gluten Free

The leaves and stem tips of cilantro are rich in numerous antioxidant flavonoids that scavenge free radicals and help prevent the onset of heart disease and cancer.

INGREDIENTS

1 bunch fresh cilantro, destemmed

2 jalapenos, sliced

4 tablespoons lime juice

2 tablespoons canola oil

1 teaspoon sea salt

½ teaspoon black pepper

Canola oil is a good source of monounsaturated fat and omega-3 fats. New research findings suggest that consuming canola oil may help to decrease abdominal fat.

DIRECTIONS

1) Place all of the ingredients in a food processor. Use the chop setting and process until it is a smooth consistency. Place in the refrigerator for up to 1 week.

Per Serving: Kcal 30, Protein 0g, Carb 1g, Fat 3g, Sodium 182mg, Dietary Fiber 1g,
Daily Values: Fiber 2%, Vitamin C 10%, Vitamin A 0%, Vitamin D 0% Potassium 2% Calcium 1%, Iron 1%

Roasted Strawberry Vinaigrette

Servings: 8 ✦ Serving Size: 2 tablespoons

Vegan, Gluten Free

In this recipe, I roast the strawberries to bring out the natural sweetness of the fruit. Combined with thyme, the herbal notes offer a great compliment to the sweet berry flavors. Canola oil has a light texture and neutral taste, which showcases the flavors of herbs, spices, and other ingredients.

INGREDIENTS

8 medium-sized strawberries, destemmed and cut in half

½ teaspoon dried thyme

Canola oil spray

½ teaspoon mustard

⅛ teaspoon sea salt

2 tablespoons red wine vinegar

1 tablespoon canola oil

Antioxidants, fiber, and phytochemicals in strawberries have been shown to reduce total cholesterol levels. Plus, the potassium found in strawberries can help control blood pressure and fight strokes.

DIRECTIONS

1) Preheat the oven to 400°F on the roast feature. In a medium-sized bowl, place the strawberries and thyme.

2) Cover a baking sheet with aluminum foil and spray with canola oil spray. Add the strawberry mixture and roast for 8 minutes. Remove from the oven and let cool for 1 minute.

3) In a food processor, place the strawberry mixture. Be sure to put any excess juices left over from the baking sheet into the processor. Add the mustard, salt, vinegar, and oil. Puree until the mixture reaches a smooth consistency.

4) Refrigerate and store for up to 1 week.

Per Serving: Kcal 22, Protein 0g, Carb 1.5g, Fat 2g, Sodium 28mg, Dietary Fiber 0g
Daily Values: Fiber 1.4%, Vitamin C 12%, Vitamin A 0%, Vitamin D 0%, Potassium 30%, Calcium 0.4%, Iron 1%

Summer Shopping List

This shopping list sets forth the ingredients that are needed only for the recipes included in the 7-day menu plans. If you choose to replace one recipe with another, please make sure to look at the recipe before shopping and buy the proper ingredients. For a downloadable version of this shopping list, visit *www.flatbelly365.com/resources*.

Produce

- ❏ 5 medium mangos
- ❏ 4 pounds strawberries
- ❏ 1 pint raspberry
- ❏ 4 cucumbers
- ❏ 1 watermelon
- ❏ 4 nectarines
- ❏ 4 large yellow zucchinis
- ❏ 3 ears of corn
- ❏ 1 pound yellow cherry tomatoes
- ❏ 1 red bell pepper
- ❏ 1 bunch celery stalks
- ❏ 1 (16 oz) package of figs
- ❏ 1 medium jicama
- ❏ 3 medium red onions
- ❏ 1 medium tomato
- ❏ 1 whole avocado
- ❏ 2 whole peaches
- ❏ 1 papaya

- ❑ 2 carrots
- ❑ 1 (9 oz) bag spinach
- ❑ 1 (5 oz) bag arugula
- ❑ 1 fennel bulb
- ❑ 1 (5 oz) bag mixed greens
- ❑ 1 bunch parsley
- ❑ 1 bunch basil
- ❑ 1 bunch mint
- ❑ 1 head garlic
- ❑ Lemon juice

Dairy and Eggs

- ❑ 1 (16 oz) container 2% plain Greek yogurt*
- ❑ 1 (8 oz) package aged Parmesan cheese
- ❑ Half dozen eggs

Pantry

- ❑ Olive oil
- ❑ Canola oil
- ❑ 1 (8.5 fl. oz) bottle white wine vinegar
- ❑ 1 (8.5 fl. oz) bottle red wine vinegar
- ❑ 1 (8 oz) bottle yellow mustard or mustard of choice
- ❑ 1 (12 oz) box red quinoa
- ❑ 1 (8 oz) bag chia seeds
- ❑ 1 (16 oz) bag almonds
- ❑ 1 (8 oz) bag sunflower seeds
- ❑ 1 (16 oz) bag chopped walnuts
- ❑ 1 (16 oz) bag pistachios

❑ 1 (32 fl. oz) container low sodium vegetable stock*

❑ 1 (15 oz) can garbanzo beans

Meats and Vegetarian Proteins

❑ 2 pounds boneless, skinless chicken breast or lean protein of choice*

❑ Other choices: White fish, canned tuna, salmon, shrimp, pork loin, sirloin steak, tofu, tempeh, and seitan

Spices

❑ Black pepper

❑ Sea salt

❑ Chili powder

❑ Dried thyme

❑ Dried basil

Other

❑ Protein powder* *(whey, soy, pea, or rice)*

Additional ingredients for 1,800 Calorie Menu only

Produce

❑ 1 medium cucumber

❑ 1 small red onion

❑ 1 pound yellow cherry tomatoes

❑ 1 whole avocado

❑ 1 green bell pepper

❑ 1 (4 oz) container aji Amarillo paste or other chili paste

❑ 1 lime

* Denotes items that need to be doubled for 1,800 calorie menu

CHAPTER 5

The 7-Day Fall Reboot

In history, fall or autumn was always linked to the time of the "harvest," when families and villages gathered to harvest grains that were planted during the summer months. If the "harvest" was big, people often held festivals to celebrate the bounty that would have to last during the coming winter months. During this season, I decided to incorporate not just the starchy vegetables, but also grains and legumes such as wild rice, oatmeal, beans, sweet potatoes, and the seasonal favorite, pumpkin, to showcase the true flavors of the season. Again, I played around with the temperatures of the recipes by using warm smoothies and adding a few more grain bowls, as well as delicious, creamy soups. A quick chart helps to identify the seasonal bounty available at grocery stores and farmers' markets.

Table 6: Seasonal Fruits and Vegetables During Fall*

Fruits	Vegetables
Apples	Artichokes
Asian pears	Arugula
Blackberries	Beets
Cactus pears	Broccoli
Cranberries	Broccoli rabe
Dates	Brussels sprouts
Figs	Cabbage
Grapefruit	Carrots
Jujubes	Cauliflower
Kiwi	Celeriac
Limes	Celery
Melons	Corn
Nectarines	Cucumbers
Olives	Eggplant
Oranges	Fennel
Peaches	Ginger root
Pears	Leeks
Persimmons	Mushrooms
Plums	Mustard greens
Pomegranates	Okra
Quince	Onions

Fruits *(continued)*	Vegetables *(continued)*
Raspberries	Parsnips
Strawberries	Peas
	Peppers (sweet and chili)
	Purslane
	Rutabaga
	Winter squash
	Sunchokes
	Sweet potatoes
	Tomatoes
	Tomatillos
	Turnips

* For a downloadable version of this table, visit www.flatbelly365.com/resources

Fall 1,300 Calorie 7-Day Menu

	Monday	Tuesday	Wednesday	Thursday
Breakfast	**1 cup** *Fall Spiced Oatmeal Bowl* (see page 94) TOPPINGS: **4 halves** walnuts **1 tablespoon** dried cranberries **1 teaspoon** chia seeds	**1 cup** *Fall Spiced Oatmeal Bowl* (see page 94) TOPPINGS: **4 halves** walnuts **1 tablespoon** dried cranberries **1 teaspoon** chia seeds	**2 cups** *Pumpkin Pie Smoothie* (see page 95) **1** hard-boiled egg	**1 cup** *Fall Spiced Oatmeal Bowl* (see page 94) TOPPINGS: **4 halves** walnuts **1 tablespoon** dried cranberries **1 teaspoon** chia seeds
Snack	**1 ounce** aged Parmesan cheese **17** grapes or fruit of choice (see Table 6)	**½ cup** applesauce **1 tablespoon** dried chia seeds	**1 ounce** aged Parmesan cheese **17** grapes or fruit of choice (see Table 6)	**½ cup** applesauce **1 tablespoon** dried chia seeds
Lunch	**1¼ cups** *Wild Rice with Stir Fry Vegetables Bowl* (see page 98) **3 oz.** boneless, skinless chicken breast, baked or grilled or protein of choice (see Table 2)	**1¼ cups** *Wild Rice with Stir Fry Vegetables Bowl* (see page 98) **3 oz.** boneless, skinless chicken breast, baked or grilled or protein of choice (see Table 2)	**2 cups** *Sweet Potato a la Paprika Bean Bowl* (see page 96) **3 oz.** boneless, skinless chicken breast, baked or grilled or protein of choice (see Table 2)	**2 cups** *Sweet Potato a la Paprika Bean Bowl* (see page 96) **3 oz.** boneless, skinless chicken breast, baked or grilled or protein of choice (see Table 2)
Snack	**3** prunes **12** almonds	**½ cup** plain 2% Greek yogurt TOPPINGS: **4 halves** walnuts **1 tablespoon** dried cranberries	**3** prunes **12** almonds	**½ cup** plain 2% Greek yogurt TOPPINGS: **4 halves** walnuts **1 tablespoon** dried cranberries
Dinner	**1½ cups** *Creamy Butternut Squash Soup* (see page 101) **3 oz.** boneless, skinless chicken breast, baked or grilled or protein of choice (see Table 2)	**1½ cups** *Smoky Tomato Soup* (see page 100) **3 oz.** boneless, skinless chicken breast, baked or grilled or protein of choice (see Table 2)	**1½ cups** *Creamy Butternut Squash Soup* (see page 101) **3 oz.** boneless, skinless chicken breast, baked or grilled or protein of choice (see Table 2)	**1½ cups** *Creamy Butternut Squash Soup* (see page 101) **3 oz.** boneless, skinless chicken breast, baked or grilled or protein of choice (see Table 2)

Fall 1,300 Calorie 7-Day Menu *(continued)*

	Friday	Saturday	Sunday
Breakfast	**2 cups** *Pumpkin Pie Smoothie* *(see page 95)* **1** hard-boiled egg	**1 cup** *Fall Spiced Oatmeal Bowl* *(see page 94)* TOPPINGS: **4 halves** walnuts **1 tablespoon** dried cranberries **1 teaspoon** chia seeds	**2 cups** *Pumpkin Pie Smoothie* *(see page 95)* **1** hard-boiled egg
Snack	**½ cup** applesauce **1 tablespoon** dried chia seeds	**1 ounce** aged Parmesan cheese **17** grapes or fruit of choice *(see Table 6)*	**½ cup** applesauce **1 tablespoon** dried chia seeds
Lunch	**1¼ cups** *Wild Rice with Stri Fry Vegetable Bowl* *(see page 98)* **3 oz.** boneless, skinless chicken breast, baked or grilled or protein of choice *(see Table 2)*	**2 cups** *Sweet Potato a la Paprika Bean Bowl* *(see page 96)* **3 oz.** boneless, skinless chicken breast, baked or grilled or protein of choice *(see Table 2)*	**1½ cups** *Creamy Butternut Squash Soup* *(see page 101)* **3 oz.** boneless, skinless chicken breast, baked or grilled or protein of choice *(see Table 2)*
Snack	**3** prunes **12** almonds	**½ cup** plain 2% Greek yogurt TOPPINGS: **4 halves** walnuts **1 tablespoon** dried cranberries	**3** prunes **12** almonds
Dinner	**2 cups** *Sweet Potato a la Paprika Bean Bowl* *(see page 96)* **3 oz.** boneless, skinless chicken breast, baked or grilled or protein of choice *(see Table 2)*	**1¼ cup** *Wild Rice with Stir Fry Vegetable Bowl* *(see page 98)* **3 oz.** boneless, skinless chicken breast, baked or grilled or protein of choice *(see Table 2)*	**1½ cups** *Smoky Tomato Soup* *(see page 100)* **3 oz.** boneless, skinless chicken breast, baked or grilled or protein of choice *(see Table 2)*

Fall 1,800 Calorie 7-Day Menu

	Monday	Tuesday	Wednesday	Thursday
Breakfast	**1 cup** *Fall Spiced Oatmeal Bowl* (see page 94) TOPPINGS: **4 halves** walnuts **1 tablespoon** dried cranberries **1 teaspoon** chia seeds or toppings of choice (see Table 3)	**1 cup** *Fall Spiced Oatmeal Bowl* (see page 94) TOPPINGS: **4 halves** walnuts **1 tablespoon** dried cranberries **1 teaspoon** chia seeds or toppings of choice (see Table 3)	**2 cups** *Pumpkin Pie Smoothie* (see page 95) **2** hard-boiled eggs	**1 cup** *Fall Spiced Oatmeal Bowl* (see page 94) TOPPINGS: **4 halves** walnuts **1 tablespoon** dried cranberries **1 teaspoon** chia seeds or toppings of choice (see Table 3)
Snack	**2 oz** aged Parmesan cheese **17** grapes or fruit of choice (see Table 6)	**1 cup** applesauce **2 tablespoons** chia seeds	**2 oz** aged Parmesan cheese **17** grapes or fruit of choice (see Table 6)	**1 cup** applesauce **2 tablespoons** dried chia seeds
Lunch	**2 cups** *Wild Rice with Stir Fry Vegetable Bowl* (see page 98) **6 oz** boneless, skinless chicken breast, baked or grilled or protein of choice (see Table 2)	**2 cups** *Wild Rice with Stir Fry Vegetable Bowl* (see page 98) **6 oz** boneless, skinless chicken breast, baked or grilled or protein of choice (see Table 2)	**2 cups** *Sweet Potato a la Paprika Bean Bowl* (see page 96) **6 oz** boneless, skinless chicken breast, baked or grilled or protein of choice (see Table 2)	**2 cups** *Sweet Potato a la Paprika Bean Bowl* (see page 96) **6 oz** boneless, skinless chicken breast, baked or grilled or protein of choice (see Table 2)
Snack	**6** prunes **18** almonds	**1 cup** plain 2% Greek yogurt TOPPINGS: **4 halves** walnuts **1 tablespoon** dried cranberries	**6** prunes **18** almonds	**1 cup** plain 2% Greek yogurt TOPPINGS: **4 halves** walnuts **1 tablespoon** dried cranberries
Dinner	**1½ cups** *Creamy Butternut Squash Soup* (see page 101) **6 oz** boneless, skinless chicken breast, baked or grilled or protein of choice (see Table 2)	**1½ cups** *Smoky Tomato Soup* (see page 100) **6 oz** boneless, skinless chicken breast, baked or grilled or protein of choice (see Table 2)	**1½ cups** *Creamy Butternut Squash Soup* (see page 101) **6 oz** boneless, skinless chicken breast, baked or grilled or protein of choice (see Table 2)	**1½ cups** *Creamy Butternut Squash Soup* (see page 101) **6 oz** boneless, skinless chicken breast, baked or grilled or protein of choice (see Table 2)

Fall 1,800 Calorie 7-Day Menu *(continued)*

	Friday	Saturday	Sunday
Breakfast	**2 cups** *Pumpkin Pie Smoothie* *(see page 95)* **2** hard-boiled eggs	**1 cup** *Fall Spiced Oatmeal Bowl* *(see page 94)* TOPPINGS: **4 halves** walnuts **1 tablespoon** dried cranberries **1 teaspoon** chia seeds or toppings of choice *(see Table 3)*	**2 cups** *Pumpkin Pie Smoothie* *(see page 95)* **2** hard-boiled eggs
Snack	**1 cup** applesauce **2 tablespoons** dried chia seeds	**2 oz** aged Parmesan cheese **17** grapes or fruit of choice *(see Table 6)*	**1 cup** applesauce **2 tablespoons** dried chia seeds
Lunch	**2 cups** *Wild Rice with Stir Fry Vegetable Bowl* *(see page 98)* **6 oz** boneless, skinless chicken breast, baked or grilled or protein of choice *(see Table 2)*	**2 cups** *Sweet Potato a la Paprika Bean Bowl* *(see page 96)* **6 oz** boneless, skinless chicken breast, baked or grilled or protein of choice *(see Table 2)*	**1½ cups** *Creamy Butternut Squash Soup* *(see page 101)* **6 oz** boneless, skinless chicken breast, baked or grilled or protein of choice *(see Table 2)*
Snack	**6** prunes **18** almonds	**1 cup** plain 2% Greek yogurt TOPPINGS: **4 halves** walnuts **1 tablespoon** dried cranberries	**6** prunes **18** almonds
Dinner	**2 cups** *Sweet Potato a la Paprika Bean Bowl* *(see page 96)* **6 oz** boneless, skinless chicken breast, baked or grilled or protein of choice *(see Table 2)*	**2 cups** *Wild Rice with Stir Fry Vegetable Bowl* *(see page 98)* **6 oz** boneless, skinless chicken breast, baked or grilled or protein of choice *(see Table 2)*	**1½ cups** *Smoky Tomato Soup* *(see page 100)* **6 oz** boneless, skinless chicken breast, baked or grilled or protein of choice *(see Table 2)*

Fall Spiced Oatmeal

Servings: 4 ✦ Serving Size: 1 cup

Vegan, Gluten Free

This isn't your traditional bland oatmeal. I combine the naturally sweet flavors of pumpkin with the subtle spice notes of the pumpkin spice blend to make this mouthwatering oatmeal dish. Pumpkin also contains beta carotene, which is a powerful antioxidant known to help promote vision and neurological functions (see the color photo page 166).

INGREDIENTS

1½ cups dry oats

2¼ cups vanilla soy or almond milk

⅛ teaspoon sea salt

¼ teaspoon pumpkin spice

½ cup pumpkin puree

When oats are ingested, they are fermented by the gut bacteria. This can improve your gut flora, which then improves your digestive health.

DIRECTIONS

1) In a medium-sized pan, place the dry oats, soy milk, salt, and pumpkin spice. Cook on medium heat until the oats are soft.

2) Add the pumpkin puree and stir. Cook for another 5 minutes until the mixture has thickened. Stir occasionally. Mix in the topping of your choice from the table on page 25 and serve.

Per Serving: Kcal 289, Protein 11 g, Carb 50 g, Fat 6 g, Sodium 308 mg, Dietary Fiber 8 g, Daily Values: Fiber 27%, Vitamin C 1%, Vitamin A 36%, Vitamin D 7%, Potassium 8%, Calcium 23%, Iron 20%

Pumpkin Pie Smoothie

Servings: 1 ✦ Serving Size: 2 cups

Vegan, Gluten Free

The crisp cool days are seeping in, and this smoothie is here to warm you up. Here is the best part of a warm pumpkin pie, but in a smoothie, to help you get a great start to your day. Pumpkin is also packed with beta carotene, which helps to promote healthy bone growth and a strong immunity defense.

INGREDIENTS

1 cup pumpkin puree

¾ cup vanilla soy milk

1 small banana

½ teaspoon cinnamon

1 scoop protein powder*
   (whey, soy, or pea)

Note: To provide 20 grams of protein.

Bananas are a good source of fructooligosaccharide, a potent prebiotic that can help promote the growth of good bacteria in the gastrointestinal tract. Bananas are the easiest way to incorporate more prebiotics into your diet.

DIRECTIONS

1) Blend all the ingredients in a blender until smooth. In a small saucepan, warm up the smoothie on medium heat. Do not boil.

Per Serving: Kcal 371, Protein 32 g, Carb 58 g, Fat 4 g, Sodium 236.0 mg, Dietary Fiber 12 g,
Daily Values: Fiber 44%, Vitamin C 23%, Vitamin A 212%, Vitamin D 0%, Potassium 23%, Calcium 35%, Iron 27%

Sweet Potato a la Paprika Bean Bowl

Servings: 4 ✦ Serving Size: 1 serving

Vegan, Gluten Free

Sweet potatoes aren't just for pie. I combine them with the smoky flavor of paprika to create a delicious spin. Mixed with black beans, this hearty dish can be eaten at any time of the day (see the color photo page 169).

INGREDIENTS

3 cups (16 oz) sweet potatoes, peeled and chopped into ½-inch squares

2 teaspoons paprika

¼ teaspoon sea salt

Canola oil spray

1 teaspoon canola oil

½ red onion, chopped

½ teaspoon garlic, crushed

1 can black beans, drained and washed

½ teaspoon cumin

½ teaspoon chili powder

¼ cup fresh cilantro, chopped

2 scallions, sliced

Even though they are known to create gas, beans are actually a gut healthy food. Beans feed the good bacteria in your gut and rev up your immune system. Also, beans are packed with fiber, which can improve weight loss by enhancing satiety.

DIRECTIONS

1) Preheat oven to 400°F.

2) In a 9 x 9 roasting pan, place the sweet potatoes, paprika, and sea salt. Spray with enough canola oil to coat the potato mixture. Toss to mix the seasonings and then place the roasting pan in the oven. Cook for 25 minutes or until the potatoes are soft.

3) Heat up a medium-sized sauté pan on medium-high heat. Place the canola oil in the pan and heat for about 2 minutes. Add the onion and garlic and sauté for 3 minutes or until the onion becomes translucent.

4) Add the beans, cumin, and chili powder. Cook for 5 minutes or until almost all the liquid has evaporated. Turn off the heat, then add the cilantro and scallions. Mix with the sweet potatoes.

Per Serving: Kcal 254, Protein 11 g, Carb 48 g, Fat 3 g, Sodium 187 mg, Dietary Fiber 13 g,
Daily Values: Fiber 46%, Vitamin C 8%, Vitamin A 82%, Vitamin D 0%, Potassium 17%, Calcium 6%, Iron 19%

Wild Rice with Stir Fry Vegetable Bowl

Servings: 4 ✦ Serving Size: 1¼ tablespoons

Vegan, Gluten Free

This rustic dish shows off the versatility of the seasonal vegetables, beyond steaming and adding them to salads. The subtleties of flavor and spice bring a whole new dimension to the season (see the color photo page 170).

INGREDIENTS for the WILD RICE

3 cups water

1 cup uncooked wild rice

½ teaspoon sea salt

INGREDIENTS for the STIR FRY

1 tablespoon canola oil

1 pound Brussels sprouts,
cut into ¼-inch pieces

½ red onion, chopped

1 bunch Swiss chard, chopped

½ teaspoon sea salt

¼ teaspoon black pepper

1 teaspoon smoked paprika

1 tablespoon tomato paste

Wild rice is an excellent source of zinc, meeting 15 percent of your Daily Value per cup, cooked. Zinc helps to strengthen immunity and the digestive system, control diabetes, reduce stress levels, and boost metabolism.

DIRECTIONS

1) *For wild rice:* In a large saucepan, bring the water to boil, then stir in the wild rice and salt. Lower the heat and simmer, covered, for 40 to 45 minutes, or just until the kernels puff open. Uncover and fluff with a fork and simmer for an additional 5 minutes. Drain any excess liquid.

2) *For stir fry vegetables:* Heat a large sauté pan on medium high heat for 1 minute. Place canola oil in the pan and heat for another minute. Add the Brussels sprouts and sauté for 5 minutes, stirring occasionally. Add the onion and sauté for 2 minutes. Finally, add the Swiss chard and sauté for another 2 minutes.

3) Add the salt, pepper, paprika, and tomato paste. Sauté for another 2 minutes while stirring.

4) In a large bowl, combine the Brussels sprout mixture and the cooked wild rice. Be sure to mix them well.

Per Serving: Kcal 225, Protein 11 g, Carb 44 g, Fat 4 g, Sodium 607 mg, Dietary Fiber 8 g,
Daily Values: Fiber 30%, Vitamin C 125%, Vitamin A 23%, Vitamin D 0%, Potassium 18%, Calcium 7%, Iron 20%

Smoky Tomato Soup

Servings: 4 ✦ Serving Size: 1½ cups

Vegan, Gluten Free

A modern twist to a timeless classic. I add artichokes to this soup to give it an extra boost of superfood goodness. Canned tomatoes contain higher levels of lycopene, a powerful phytonutrient that is known to promote prostate health. With this soup, you can warm your heart and feel healthy (see the color photo page 168).

INGREDIENTS

1 tablespoon olive oil

1 medium red onion, chopped

2 (28 oz) cans San Marzano or other brand plum tomatoes

2 medium-sized red bell pepper, chopped

1 can artichoke hearts, in water, chopped

1 cup low sodium vegetable or chicken stock

2 teaspoons dried basil

2 teaspoons paprika

1 teaspoon sea salt

1 tablespoon fresh basil, chopped

One teaspoon of paprika has 4 percent of the recommended daily vitamin intake of B6. Like most B vitamins, B6 is a coenzyme that helps maintain an efficient metabolism.

DIRECTIONS

1) Heat up a large saucepan on medium-high heat for 2 minutes. Add the oil and the onion. Sauté for about 5 minutes or until the onion becomes translucent. Add the tomatoes, bell peppers, and artichoke hearts. Stir and cook for 5 more minutes.

2) Add the stock, dried basil, paprika, and sea salt. Bring to a boil and then lower the heat to low. Cover and let simmer for 25 to 30 minutes.

3) Remove from the heat, add the fresh basil, stir, and let cool for 5 minutes. Once cooled, transfer the soup to a blender or use a hand blender and puree until it is a smooth consistency.

Per Serving: Kcal 177, Protein 7 g, Carb 32 g, Fat 5 g, Sodium 991 mg, Dietary Fiber 14 g,
Daily Values: Fiber 50%, Vitamin C 115%, Vitamin A 16%, Vitamin D 0%, Potassium 23%, Calcium 8%, Iron 22%

Creamy Butternut Squash Soup

Servings: 6 ✦ Serving Size: 1 cup

Vegan, Gluten Free

The fall season has a variety of different squash and root vegetables. I combine a few of these seasonal superfoods to create a delicious, creamy soup to warm your heart. Even though the soup is "creamy," it does not contain any cream. Rather, "creamy" refers to the smooth texture of the soup (see the color photo page 165).

INGREDIENTS

1 tablespoon olive oil

1 medium red onion, chopped

1½ cups carrots, chopped

7 cups butternut squash, chopped

½-inch nub of ginger, sliced thinly

3 cups low sodium vegetable stock or chicken stock

1 teaspoon sea salt

½ teaspoon black pepper

Ginger has been shown to support the body's natural defenses against diseases by activating T-cells, which are capable of destroying infected cells.

DIRECTIONS

1) Heat up a large saucepan on medium-high heat for 2 minutes. Place the oil and the onion in the pan. Sauté the onion for about 5 minutes or until it becomes translucent. Add the carrots, squash, and ginger. Stir and cook for 5 minutes.

2) Add the stock, sea salt, and pepper. Bring to a boil and then lower the heat to low. Cover and let simmer for 25 to 30 minutes.

3) Remove from the heat and let the mixture cool for 5 minutes. Once cooled, transfer to a blender or use a hand blender and puree until the soup has a smooth consistency.

Per Serving: Kcal 115, Protein 3 g, Carb 24 g, Fat 3 g, Sodium 594 mg, Dietary Fiber 4 g,
Daily Values: Fiber 16%, Vitamin C 42%, Vitamin A 125%, Vitamin D 0%, Potassium 15%, Calcium 8%, Iron 8%

Moroccan Lamb Stew

Servings: 8 ✦ Serving Size: 1 cup

Gluten Free

This stew was inspired by chef dietitian Katie Cavuto while I accompanied her in a culinary lamb tour. It has a hearty blend of flavors, such as cinnamon, cumin, and coriander, so it's perfect for the fall season. It also provides a good source of fiber to maintain your gut health (see the color photo page 167).

INGREDIENTS:

1 tablespoon ground cumin

1 tablespoon ground coriander

1 teaspoon fennel seeds

½ teaspoon sea salt

½ teaspoon ground pepper

3 pounds trimmed leg of lamb, cut into 1½- to 2-inch pieces

2 tablespoons canola oil, divided

1 large onion, finely chopped

4 cloves garlic, minced

1 tablespoon grated ginger

1 tablespoon tomato paste

½ cup red wine

3 cups low-sodium chicken broth

1 (15.5 ounce) can garbanzo beans (chickpeas), drained

1 (14.5 ounce) can diced canned tomatoes and their juice

1 cup carrots, sliced

2 cinnamon sticks

2 teaspoons (packed) grated lemon peel

Lean lamb is a nutrient-packed powerhouse and a source of healthy, unsaturated fats. Forty percent of the fat in lean lamb is heart healthy monounsaturated fat.

1 cup prunes, pitted

2 tablespoons chopped fresh cilantro

¼ cup toasted pine nuts

DIRECTIONS:

1) Mix the cumin, coriander, fennel seeds, salt, and pepper in a bowl. Add lamb and toss to coat.

2) Heat 2 tablespoons of oil in heavy large stock pot or Dutch oven over medium-high heat. Working in batches, add half the lamb to the pot and cook until browned on all sides, turning occasionally for 6-8 minutes. Once the lamb is browned, remove it from the pan and repeat with the remaining lamb. Set the lamb aside.

3) Add onion, garlic, ginger, and tomato paste to the pot. Reduce heat to medium; sauté until onion is soft, about 5 minutes.

4) Turn the heat up to medium high and add the wine, deglazing the pan by scraping up any bits.

5) Once the pan is deglazed, after about 1 minute, add the broth, garbanzo beans, tomatoes, carrots, cinnamon sticks, and lemon zest. Return the lamb to the pot and bring to a boil. Reduce heat to low, cover, and simmer until lamb is just tender, about 45 minutes.

6) Add prunes and stir. Uncover and simmer until sauce thickens enough to coat spoon, about 15–20 minutes.

7) Season with salt and pepper to taste. Sprinkle with cilantro and pine nuts and serve.

Per Serving: Kcal 509, Protein 52 g, Carb 29 g, Fat 19 g, Sodium 575 mg, Dietary Fiber 5 g,
Daily Values: Fiber 20%, Vitamin C 13%, Vitamin A 18%, Vitamin D 8% Potassium 12% Calcium 4%, Iron 10%

Fall Shopping List

This shopping list contains the ingredients that are needed for only the recipes included in the 7-day menu plans. If you choose to replace one recipe with another, please make sure to look at the recipe before shopping and buy the proper ingredients. For a downloadable version of this shopping list, visit *www.flatbelly365.com/resources.*

Produce

❏ 2 red bell peppers

❏ 3 carrots

❏ 1 medium butternut squash

❏ 1 pound Brussels sprouts*

❏ 5 red onions

❏ 3 small bananas

❏ 1 (1 lb) bag grapes

❏ 2 pounds sweet potatoes (yellow or orange)*

❏ 1 bunch Swiss chard*

❏ 2 bunch scallions

❏ 1 nub fresh ginger

❏ 1 bunch fresh cilantro

❏ 1 head garlic

❏ 1 bunch fresh basil

Dairy and Eggs

❏ 1 quart container almond or soy milk, unsweetened*

❏ 1 (8 oz) package aged Parmesan cheese

❑ 1 (16 oz) container 2% plain Greek yogurt*

❑ 1 half dozen eggs

Pantry

❑ Canola oil spray

❑ Canola oil

❑ Olive oil

❑ 1 (32 fl. oz) container low sodium vegetable stock or chicken stock

❑ 2 (28 oz) cans San Marzano or other brand plum tomatoes

❑ 1 (6 oz) can tomato paste

❑ 1 (15 oz) can pumpkin puree*

❑ 1 (15 oz) can artichoke hearts, in water

❑ 2 (15 oz) cans black beans*

❑ 1 (16 oz) bag dried cranberries

❑ 1 (16 oz) bag chopped walnuts

❑ 1 (8 oz) bag chia seeds

❑ 1 (16 oz) bag almonds

❑ 1 (32 oz) jar unsweetened applesauce

❑ 1 (16 oz) bag Sunsweet Amaz!ng Prunes

❑ 1 (18 oz) container dry oats

❑ 1 (2 lb) bag wild rice

❑ 1 container protein powder of choice

Meats or Vegetarian Proteins

❑ 2 pounds boneless, skinless chicken breast or lean protein of choice*

❑ Other choices: White fish, canned tuna, salmon, shrimp, pork loin, sirloin steak, tofu, tempeh, and seitan

Spices

❑ Sea salt

❑ Black pepper

❑ Pumpkin spice

❑ Cinnamon

❑ Chili powder

❑ Cumin

❑ Smoked paprika

❑ Dried basil

Other

❑ Protein powder* *(whey, soy, pea, or rice)*

* Denotes items that need to be doubled for 1,800 calorie menu

CHAPTER 6

The 7-Day Winter Reboot

Winter is known for its harsh, cold temperatures, short days, and long nights. It is plain to see why most people stay indoors and consume warm, if not hot, meals throughout the day. But just because these are the winter months, it doesn't mean that there are no seasonal superfoods. In fact, most of the common superfoods we know, such as apples, cauliflower, and broccoli, flourish in the winter months. With these recipes, I decided to bring comfort to a new level by providing chunky soups, warm salads, hot smoothies, and different grain bowls to keep you warm throughout the season. A quick chart identifies the seasonal bounty available at grocery stores and farmers' markets.

Table 7: Seasonal Fruits and Vegetables During Winter*

Fruits	Vegetables
Apples	Beets
Cherimoya	Bok choy
Citron	Broccoli
Grapefruit	Broccoli rabe
Kumquats	Brussels sprouts
Lemons	Cabbage
Limes	Carrots
Mandarins	Cauliflower
Oranges	Chicory
Pomegranates	Dandelion greens
Pomelos	Fava beans
	Fennel
	Kale
	Leeks
	Mushrooms
	Olives
	Parsnips
	Pea shoots
	Radishes
	Rutabaga
	Sunchokes

Fruits *(continued)*	Vegetables *(continued)*
	Swiss chard
	Taro root
	Turnips

* For a downloadable version of this table, visit www.flatbelly365.com/resources

Winter 1,300 Calorie 7-Day Menu

	Monday	Tuesday	Wednesday	Thursday
Breakfast	**1 cup** *Apple Spiced Oatmeal* (see page 116) TOPPINGS: **8 halves** walnuts	**2 cups** *Hot Apple Cinnamon Smoothie* (see page 114)	**2 cups** *Hot Chocolate Smoothie* (see page 115)	**1 cup** *Apple Spiced Oatmeal* (see page 116) TOPPINGS: **8 halves** walnuts
Snack	**1 medium** apple or fruit of choice (see Table 7)	**1 medium** apple or fruit of choice (see Table 7)	**1 medium** apple or fruit of choice (see Table 7)	**1 medium** apple or fruit of choice (see Table 7)
Lunch	**1 cup** *Cannellini Chicken Sausage Bowl* (see page 118) **3½ cups** mixed greens salad with lemon juice and salt (optional)	**1 cup** *Cannellini Chicken Sausage Bowl* (see page 118) **3½ cups** mixed greens salad with lemon juice and salt (optional)	**1** *Warm Candied Onion Spinach Salad* (see page 117) **3 oz** boneless, skinless chicken breast, baked or grilled or protein of choice (see Table 2)	**1 cup** *Cannellini Sausage Bowl* (see page 118) **3½ cups** mixed greens salad with lemon juice and salt (optional)
Snack	**1** orange or fruit of choice (see Table 7) **12** almonds	**¼ cup** Kefir Hummus (see page 124) **1 cup** carrot sticks	**1 oz** aged Parmesan cheese **1** orange or fruit of choice (see Table 7)	**1** orange or fruit of choice (see Table 7) **12** almonds
Dinner	**2 cups** *Cauliflower Walnut Soup* (see page 122) **3 oz** boneless, skinless chicken breast, baked or grilled or protein of choice (see Table 2)	**2 cups** *Cauliflower Walnut Soup* (see page 122) **3 oz** boneless, skinless chicken breast, baked or grilled or protein of choice (see Table 2)	**1½ cups** *Barley Eggplant Bowl* (see page 120) **3 oz** boneless, skinless chicken breast, baked or grilled or protein of choice (see Table 2)	**2 cups** *Cauliflower Walnut Soup* (see page 122) **3 oz** boneless, skinless chicken breast, baked or grilled or protein of choice (see Table 2)

Winter 1,300 Calorie 7-Day Menu *(continued)*

	Friday	Saturday	Sunday
Breakfast	**1 cup** *Apple Spiced Oatmeal* *(see page 116)* TOPPINGS: **8 halves** walnuts	**1 cup** *Apple Spiced Oatmeal* *(see page 116)* TOPPINGS: **8 halves** walnuts	**2 cups** *Hot Chocolate Smoothie* *(see page 115)*
Snack	**1 medium** apple or fruit of choice *(see Table 7)*	**1 medium** apple or fruit of choice *(see Table 7)*	**1 medium** apple or fruit of choice *(see Table 7)*
Lunch	**1½ cups** *Barley Eggplant Bowl* *(see page 120)* **3 oz** boneless, skinless chicken breast, baked or grilled or protein of choice *(see Table 2)*	**1** *Warm Candied Onion Spinach Salad* *(see page 117)* **3 oz** boneless, skinless chicken breast, baked or grilled or protein of choice *(see Table 2)*	**1½ cups** *Barley Eggplant Bowl* *(see page 120)* **3 oz** boneless, skinless chicken breast, baked or grilled or protein of choice *(see Table 2)*
Snack	**¼ cup** Kefir Hummus *(see page 124)* **1 cup** carrot sticks	**1 oz** aged Parmesan cheese **1 orange** or fruit of choice *(see Table 7)*	**¼ cup** Kefir Hummus *(see page 124)* **1 cup** carrot sticks
Dinner	**2 cups** *Cauliflower Walnut Soup* *(see page 122)* **3 oz** boneless, skinless chicken breast, baked or grilled or protein of choice *(see Table 2)*	**1 cup** *Cannellini Chicken Sausage Bowl* *(see page 118)* **3½ cups** mixed greens salad with lemon juice and salt *(optional)*	**1** *Warm Candied Onion Spinach Salad* *(see page 117)* **3 oz** boneless, skinless chicken breast, baked or grilled or protein of choice *(see Table 2)*

Winter 1,800 Calorie 7-Day Menu

	Monday	Tuesday	Wednesday	Thursday
Breakfast	**1 cup** *Apple Spiced Oatmeal* (see page 116) TOPPINGS: **8** halves walnuts	**2 cups** *Hot Apple Cinnamon Smoothie* (see page 114)	**2 cups** *Hot Chocolate Smoothie* (see page 115)	**1 cup** *Apple Spiced Oatmeal* (see page 116) TOPPINGS: **8** halves walnuts
Snack	**1 medium** apple or fruit of choice (see Table 7) **18** almonds	**1 medium** apple or fruit of choice (see Table 7) **18** almonds	**1 medium** apple or fruit of choice (see Table 7) **18** almonds	**1 medium** apple or fruit of choice (see Table 7) **18** almonds
Lunch	**1** *Warm Candied Onion Spinach Salad* (see page 117) **6 oz.** boneless, skinless chicken breast, baked or grilled or protein of choice (see Table 2)	**1½ cups** *Cannellini Chicken Sausage Bowl* (see page 118) **3½ cups** mixed greens salad with lemon juice and salt	**1½ cups** *Cannellini Chicken Sausage Bowl* (see page 118) **3½ cups** mixed greens salad with lemon juice and salt	**1** *Warm Candied Onion Spinach Salad* (see page 117) **6 oz.** boneless, skinless chicken breast, baked or grilled or protein of choice (see Table 2)
Snack	**1** orange or fruit of choice (see Table 7) **12** halves walnuts	**¼ cup** Kefir Hummus (see page 124) **1 cup** carrot sticks	**2 ounces** aged Parmesan cheese **1** orange or fruit of choice (see Table 7)	**1** orange or fruit of choice (see Table 7) **12** halves walnuts
Dinner	**2 cups** *Cauliflower Walnut Soup* (see page 122) **6 oz.** boneless, skinless chicken breast, baked or grilled or protein of choice (see Table 2)	**2 cups** *Cauliflower Walnut Soup* (see page 122) **6 oz.** boneless, skinless chicken breast, baked or grilled or protein of choice (see Table 2)	**1½ cups** *Barley Eggplant Bowl* (see page 120) **6 oz.** boneless, skinless chicken breast, baked or grilled or protein of choice (see Table 2)	**2 cups** *Cauliflower Walnut Soup* (see page 122) **6 oz.** boneless, skinless chicken breast, baked or grilled or protein of choice (see Table 2)

Winter 1,800 Calorie 7-Day Menu *(continued)*

	Friday	Saturday	Sunday
Breakfast	**1 cup** *Apple Spiced Oatmeal* *(see page 116)* TOPPINGS: **8** halves walnuts	**1 cup** *Apple Spiced Oatmeal* *(see page 116)* TOPPINGS: **8** halves walnuts	**2 cups** *Hot Chocolate Smoothie* *(see page 115)*
Snack	**1 medium** apple or fruit of choice *(see Table 7)* **18** almonds	**1 medium** apple or fruit of choice *(see Table 7)* **18** almonds	**1 medium** apple or fruit of choice *(see Table 7)* **18** almonds
Lunch	**1½ cups** *Barley Eggplant Bowl* *(see page 120)* **6 oz.** boneless, skinless chicken breast, baked or grilled or protein of choice *(see Table 2)*	**1** *Warm Candied Onion Spinach Salad* *(see page 117)* **6 oz.** boneless, skinless chicken breast, baked or grilled or protein of choice *(see Table 2)*	**2 cups** *Cauliflower Walnut Soup* *(see page 122)* **6 oz.** boneless, skinless chicken breast, baked or grilled or protein of choice *(see Table 2)*
Snack	**¼ cup** Kefir Hummus *(see page 124)* **1 cup** carrot sticks	**2 ounces** aged Parmesan cheese **1** orange or fruit of choice *(see Table 7)*	**¼ cup** Kefir Hummus *(see page 124)* **1 cup** carrot sticks
Dinner	**1½ cups** *Barley Eggplant Bowl* *(see page 120)* **6 oz.** boneless, skinless chicken breast, baked or grilled or protein of choice *(see Table 2)*	**1½ cups** *Barley Eggplant Bowl* *(see page 120)* **6 oz.** boneless, skinless chicken breast, baked or grilled or protein of choice *(see Table 2)*	**1** *Warm Candied Onion Spinach Salad* *(see page 117)* **6 oz.** boneless, skinless chicken breast, baked or grilled or protein of choice *(see Table 2)*

Hot Apple Cinnamon Smoothie

Servings: 1 ✦ Serving Size: 2 cups

Vegan, Gluten Free

Cinnamon is a spice that is used widely but hardly understood. It has anti-inflammatory and heart-healthy properties. Combined with the sweet flavors of apple, this warm smoothie is sure to get you ready for the day (see the color photo page 174).

INGREDIENTS

½ cup unsweetened apple sauce

¼ cup dry oatmeal

¼ teaspoon cinnamon powder

1 cup vanilla soy milk, or other milk of choice

1 scoop protein powder* *(whey, soy, pea, or rice)*

* *Note: To provide 20 grams of protein.*

Seasoning a high carbohydrate food with cinnamon can help prevent a spike in your blood sugar levels. Cinnamon slows the rate of gastric emptying after meals and steadies the rise in blood sugar levels after eating.

DIRECTIONS

1) Place all the ingredients in a blender and puree until the smoothie reaches your desired consistency.

2) Place the smoothie in a small saucepan on medium-high heat for 1 to 2 minutes. Do not boil.

Per Serving: Kcal 329, Protein 32 g, Carb 41 g, Fat 5 g, Sodium 284 mg, Dietary Fiber 6 g,
Daily Values: Fiber 20%, Vitamin C 29%, Vitamin A 0%, Vitamin D 0%, Potassium 7%, Calcium 36%, Iron 14%

Hot Chocolate Smoothie

Servings: 1 ✦ Serving Size: 2 cups

Vegan, Gluten Free

This isn't your normal hot chocolate. The sweetness of the banana balances the bitter notes of the cacao, making it an amazing smoothie for the winter. The cacao used here is jam-packed with flavonoids that help promote brain health.

INGREDIENTS

¼ cup dry rolled oats

1 small banana

1 tablespoon cacao powder

1 cup vanilla soy milk, or other milk of choice

1 scoop protein powder* *(whey, soy, pea, or rice)*

* *Note: To provide 20 grams of protein.*

Cacao is a natural appetite suppressant, so it can help reduce food cravings and aid in weight loss.

DIRECTIONS

1) Place all the ingredients in a blender and puree until the smoothie reaches your desired consistency.

2) Place the smoothie in a small saucepan on medium-high heat for 1 to 2 minutes. Do not boil.

Per Serving: Kcal 392, Protein 34 g, Carb 57 g, Fat 6 g, Sodium 283 mg, Dietary Fiber 9 g,
Daily Values: Fiber 31%, Vitamin C 11%, Vitamin A 0%, Vitamin D 25%, Potassium 16%, Calcium 36%, Iron 18%

Apple Spiced Oatmeal

Servings: 4 ✦ Serving Size: 1 cup

Vegan, Gluten Free

Apple and spice, and everything nice. I use both cinnamon and clove to balance the natural sweetness of the applesauce.

INGREDIENTS

3 cups water

2 cinnamon sticks

3 cloves

¼ teaspoon sea salt

2 cups dry oats

1 cup applesauce, unsweetened

½ teaspoon cinnamon powder

Research suggests that the beta-glucans found in oats are a type of fiber that can improve blood glucose control, insulin resistance, and cholesterol levels.

DIRECTIONS

1) Place the water in a saucepan with the cinnamon sticks, cloves, and salt. Bring to a boil and simmer for 5 minutes.

2) Add the oats and cook for 4 to 5 minutes.

3) Remove the cinnamon sticks and cloves.

4) Add the applesauce and cinnamon powder. Stir until it is mixed well. Set aside and let cool. Feel free to mix in your topping of choice from the list on page 25 and then serve.

Per Serving: Kcal 332, Protein 13 g, Carb 59 g, Fat 6 g, Sodium 114 mg, Dietary Fiber 9 g,
Daily Values: Fiber 34%, Vitamin C 1%, Vitamin A 0%, Vitamin D 0%, Potassium 8%, Calcium 4%, Iron 22%

Warm Candied Onion Spinach Salad

Servings: 1 ✦ Serving Size: 1 salad

Vegan, Gluten Free

Making a warm salad may sound odd, but the result is delicious. Cooking the onions with the balsamic really makes the sweetness of this salad come alive. The walnuts also lend their nutty flavor and brain-boosting goodness (see the color photo page 175).

INGREDIENTS

2 teaspoons olive oil

1 medium red onion, cut into ½-inch slices

8 walnut halves (1 ounce), roughly chopped

1 tablespoon balsamic vinegar

½ teaspoon sea salt

6 basil leaves, cut into ribbons

3 cups baby spinach

1 cup cherry tomatoes, halved

Spinach is a great source of the carotenoids lutein and zeaxanthin, two potent anti-inflammatory phytonutrients. Spinach is also packed with magnesium, iron, vitamin K, vitamin E, vitamin A, calcium, and potassium.

DIRECTIONS

1) Heat a medium-sized sauté pan on medium heat for 1 minute. Place the olive oil and onions in the pan and sauté for about 3 minutes, or until the onions become translucent.

2) Add the walnuts and cook for an additional 2 minutes.

3) Add the balsamic vinegar and salt and lower to a medium low heat. Cook for 2 minutes. Add the basil, stir, and set aside.

4) In a separate bowl, mix the spinach and cherry tomatoes together. Add the warm vegetables and mix well.

Per Serving: Kcal 297, Protein 8 g, Carb 26g, Fat 20g, Sodium 969g, Dietary Fiber 7g,
Daily Values: Fiber 26%, Vitamin C 65%, Vitamin A 56%, Vitamin D 0%, Potassium 25%, Calcium 12%, Iron 22%

Cannellini Chicken Sausage Bowl

Servings: 4 ✦ Serving Size: 1 cup

Gluten Free

Using canned beans during the winter is one of the easiest and quickest ways to add protein and fiber into your diet. This soup is a delicious combination of chicken sausage, cannellini beans, and vegetables to make for a hearty meal (see the color photo page 171).

INGREDIENTS

1 tablespoon canola oil

1 medium red onion, sliced

1 cup carrots, sliced

½ cup celery, diced

1 teaspoon sea salt

¼ teaspoon black pepper

4 (85 g) chicken sausage links, sliced *(or vegetarian sausage)*

2 (15.5 oz) cans cannellini beans, rinsed

1 (14.5 oz) can diced tomatoes

½ teaspoon Italian seasoning

Canola oil has the least amount of saturated fat of all common oils and is free of trans fat and cholesterol. It also has the most omega-3 fats of any cooking oil and is a good source of vitamin E.

DIRECTIONS

1) Heat oil in large pan and sauté onion on medium heat until translucent.

2) Add the carrots, celery, salt, and pepper and cook until tender.

3) Raise the temperature to medium heat. Add the chicken sausage and cook for 8 minutes or until the sausage begins to brown.

4) Add the cannellini beans, diced tomatoes, and Italian seasoning. Let it simmer for 5 minutes.

Per Serving: Kcal 464, Protein 33 g, Carb 61 g, Fat 11 g, Sodium 1190 mg, Dietary Fiber 13 g,
Daily Values: Fiber 47%, Vitamin C 14%, Vitamin A 30%, Vitamin D 0%, Potassium 29%, Calcium 17%, Iron 50%

Ginger-Cilantro Chicken Soup

Servings: 7 ✦ Serving Size: 2½ cups

Gluten Free

This soup is near and dear to my heart as a twist on a favorite soup from my childhood. Ginger has a myriad of health benefits, including immune-boosting abilities. This soup is perfect for warming you up on a cold winter day (see the color photo page 173).

INGREDIENTS

1 whole chicken

16 cups chicken broth

1 tablespoon minced ginger

1 cup carrots, sliced

1 cup celery, sliced

1 red onion, quartered

½ cup brown rice, raw

salt and pepper, to taste

½ cup fresh cilantro, chopped

Ginger is known to have anticancer properties, which are attributed to the phytonutrient gingerol, a natural chemical that is found in large amounts in raw ginger.

DIRECTIONS

1) Remove the skin from the whole chicken. Make sure to cut the chicken breast in half. In total, you should have 8 pieces, which include two drumsticks, two thighs, and four chicken breasts. Wings are optional to keep.

2) In a large soup pot put the chicken, water, ginger, carrots, celery, onion, and rice.

3) Heat and simmer, uncovered, for about 30 to 40 minutes or until the chicken meat falls off the bones (skim off foam every so often) and the rice is soft.

4) Season the soup with salt and pepper, to taste.

5) Once the soup is ready, throw in the cilantro.

Per Serving: Kcal 199, Protein 22 g, Carb 14 g, Fat 6 g, Sodium 88 mg, Dietary Fiber 2 g,
Daily Values: Fiber 6%, Vitamin C 5%, Vitamin A 18%, Vitamin D 1%, Potassium 7%, Calcium 2%, Iron 7%

Barley Eggplant Bowl

Servings: 4 ✦ Serving Size: 1½ cups

Vegan

Believe it or not, barley is a superfood. This ancient grain is high in both soluble and insoluble fiber, which helps promote a healthy digestive tract, helps metabolize fat, and lowers cholesterol. Combine it with tomato and eggplant for a delicious and refreshing twist.

INGREDIENTS

1 cup dry hulled barley (or farro)

1 tablespoon canola oil

1 medium red onion, chopped

2 tablespoons tomato paste

1½ teaspoons sea salt

1 pound 7 oz (8 cups) of Chinese eggplant or other eggplant, sliced and quartered

½ cup vegetable broth

2 teaspoons smoked paprika

2 teaspoons red wine vinegar

1 cup fresh basil, sliced into ribbons

Eggplants are rich in the phytonutrient nasunin, which is a potent antioxidant and free radical scavenger. It has been shown to protect cell membranes from damage.

DIRECTIONS

1) Place the barley and 6 cups of water in a medium-sized saucepan. Bring both to a boil on high heat and then lower the temperature to a low simmer. Cover and cook the barley for about 35 to 40 minutes. Barley is done when it is soft and chewy. If there is water left, drain out the excess water. Set the barley aside and let it cool.

2) Heat a large sauté pan on medium-high heat for 2 minutes. Place the canola oil in the pan and heat for another minute. Add the onion and sauté the onion for 2 minutes. Add the tomato paste and salt and cook for another minute.

3) Add the eggplant and cook for about 3 minutes and then add the vegetable broth and paprika. Stir continuously and cook for another 10 minutes.

4) Add the red wine vinegar, stir, and cook for another 2 minutes.

5) Add the basil and barley and stir to make sure the eggplant and barley are well mixed. Serve.

Per Serving: Kcal 259, Protein 8 g, Carb 49 g, Fat 5 g, Sodium 836 mg, Dietary Fiber 14 g,
Daily Values: Fiber 51%, Vitamin C 10%, Vitamin A 7%, Vitamin D 0%, Potassium 16%, Calcium 5%, Iron 16%

Cauliflower Walnut Soup

Servings: 5 ✦ Serving Size: 1½ cups

Vegan, Gluten Free

Cauliflower is one of the most popular vegetables in the winter due to its versatility. I love caramelizing it to bring out the natural sugars and to concentrate the flavors. I add walnuts to give this soup an extra health boost of omega-3 fats (see the color photo page 172).

INGREDIENTS

2 heads of cauliflower, chopped

2 tablespoons fresh thyme, chopped

Canola oil spray

1 tablespoon canola oil

1 medium red onion, chopped

1 teaspoon garlic, crushed

½ cup walnuts

6 cups low sodium vegetable or chicken stock

1½ teaspoons sea salt

½ teaspoon black pepper

What makes walnuts unique among other nuts is that they have the highest amount of omega-3 fats, with 2.5 grams per serving. Research has shown that eating walnuts can help reduce belly fat and is associated with better memory, better brain function, and even boosting your mood.

DIRECTIONS

1) Preheat oven to 400°F.

2) In a 9 x 9 roasting pan, place the cauliflower and thyme and spray them with the canola oil spray. Spray enough oil to coat the cauliflower. Place the cauliflower mixture in the oven and roast for 25 minutes. Once it is done, remove from the oven and set aside.

3) Heat up a large saucepan on medium-high heat for 2 minutes. Place the oil, onion, and garlic in the pan. Sauté for about 3 minutes. Add the walnuts and sauté for an additional 2 minutes.

4) Add the cauliflower mixture, stock, sea salt, and black pepper. Bring to a boil and then reduce the heat to low. Cover and let simmer for 15 minutes.

5) Remove from the heat and let cool for 5 minutes. Once cooled, transfer to a blender or use a hand blender and puree until it is a smooth consistency.

Per Serving: Kcal 193, Protein 7 g, Carb 19 g, Fat 12 g, Sodium 1558 mg, Dietary Fiber 6 g,
Daily Values: Fiber 21%, Vitamin C 127%, Vitamin A 4%, Vitamin D 0%, Potassium 17%, Calcium 6%, Iron 16%

Kefir Hummus

Servings: 6 ✦ Serving Size: ¼ cup

Vegetarian, Gluten Free

Hummus is a great dish because it has the right amount of carbohydrates and protein. Adding kefir gives the hummus a tangy flavor and provides a probiotic boost. The garbanzo beans provide prebiotic fibers. This hummus is ideal for gut health.

INGREDIENTS

1 (15.5 oz) can garbanzo beans, drained

½ cup kefir, plain, unsweetened

1 tablespoon lemon juice

¼ teaspoon garlic powder

¼ teaspoon black pepper

½ teaspoon sea salt

Garbanzo beans are an excellent source of dietary fiber, which can help with digestive health. They also pack magnesium, potassium, and iron.

DIRECTIONS

1) Place the ingredients in a blender and puree until they reach a smooth consistency.

Per Serving: Kcal 77, Protein 5.4 g, Carb 11 g, Fat 2 g, Sodium 358 mg, Dietary Fiber 3 g,
Daily Values: Fiber 12%, Vitamin C 1%, Vitamin A 1%, Vitamin D 0%, Potassium 3%, Calcium 4%, Iron 5%

Winter Shopping List

This shopping list contains the ingredients that are needed for only the recipes included in the 7-day menu plans. If you choose to replace one recipe with another, please make sure to look at the recipe before shopping and buy the proper ingredients. For a downloadable version of this shopping list, visit *www.flatbelly365.com/resources*.

Fruits and Vegetables:

- ❑ 1 bunch celery stalks
- ❑ 7 medium onions
- ❑ 1 (9 oz) bag baby spinach
- ❑ 2 heads cauliflower
- ❑ 6 carrots
- ❑ 3 pounds cherry tomatoes
- ❑ 2 pounds Chinese eggplant or other eggplant
- ❑ 3 oranges
- ❑ 7 medium apples
- ❑ 2 small bananas
- ❑ 1 small bag carrot sticks
- ❑ 2 small lemons
- ❑ 2 (5 oz) bags mixed greens
- ❑ 1 nub fresh ginger
- ❑ 1 head garlic
- ❑ 1 bunch fresh cilantro
- ❑ 1 bunch basil
- ❑ 1 bunch fresh thyme

Dairy and Eggs

❑ 1 quart container almond or soy milk, unsweetened

❑ 1 (8 oz) package aged Parmesan cheese

❑ 1 (32 oz) bottle plain kefir

Pantry

❑ 1 (18 oz) container dry oats

❑ 1 (2 lb) bag brown rice

❑ 1 (26 oz) bag dry hulled barley

❑ Canola oil

❑ Canola oil spray

❑ Olive oil

❑ 1 (8.5 fl. oz) bottle balsamic vinegar

❑ 1 (8.5 fl. oz) red wine vinegar

❑ 1 (16 oz) bag chopped walnuts

❑ 1 (16 oz) bag almonds

❑ 1 (8 oz) bag cacao powder

❑ 1 (6 oz) can tomato paste

❑ 1 (32 fl. oz) container low sodium chicken stock

❑ 2 (32 fl. oz) containers low sodium vegetable stock

❑ 1 (24 oz) jar unsweetened applesauce

❑ 2 (15 oz) cans cannellini beans

❑ 1 (15 oz) can garbanzo beans

Meats and Vegetarian Proteins

❑ 1 pound chicken sausage links

❑ 1 whole chicken

❑ 2 pounds boneless, skinless chicken breast or lean protein of choice*

❑ Other choices: White fish, canned tuna, salmon, shrimp, pork loin, sirloin steak, tofu, tempeh, and seitan

Spices

❑ Italian seasoning

❑ Cinnamon sticks

❑ Cinnamon powder

❑ Sea salt

❑ Basil

❑ Black pepper

❑ Smoked paprika

❑ Cloves

❑ Chili powder

Other

❑ Protein powder* *(whey, soy, pea, or rice)*

* Denotes items that need to be doubled for 1,800 calorie menu

CHAPTER 7

Staples, Sides, and Desserts for All Seasons

Assorted Fermented Vegetables

Yield: 4 (24 oz.) Mason jars ✦ Sevings: 12 ✦ Serving Size: 1 cup

Vegan, Gluten Free

Making your own fermented vegetables is quite easy. The best thing about doing this is that the vegetables can last you a month. It is important to know that you must use filtered water, not tap water. The chlorine in tap water will kill the probiotics. Also, make sure you use the correct salt and refrain from using vinegar. Ionized salt and vinegar will prevent the fermentation process that is necessary for the good bacteria to flourish. If you choose to buy a supermarket brand, make sure you purchase items that are not pickled with vinegar. More than likely, these fermented vegetables will be found in the refrigerator section of your grocery store.

INGREDIENTS for the SEASONING

4 tablespoons whole peppercorn

4 teaspoons red chili pepper

2 teaspoons celery seeds

2 teaspoons oregano

20 garlic cloves, slightly crushed

1 bunch dill

The fermentation process of vegetables enables the growth of the probiotic lactobacillus and bifidobacterium. Therefore, adding fermented vegetables to your diet will not only increase your probiotics but also your vegetable intake.

INGREDIENTS for the VEGETABLES

5 carrots, cut lengthwise

5 cucumbers, cut lengthwise

1 red onion, sliced

1 red bell pepper, cut lengthwise

¼ red cabbage, sliced

2 cups cauliflower florets, small dice

INGREDIENTS for the BRINE

8 cups filtered water

8 teaspoons sea salt or Himalayan salt

DIRECTIONS

1) In each Mason jar, evenly distribute the seasonings. For the garlic, make sure there are five cloves per jar. For the dill, remove the majority of the stem and distribute evenly.

2) For the vegetables, you can combine them and then evenly distribute them or place them in whatever pairing you like.

3) In a separate container, combine the water and salt and stir, making sure the salt is dissolved. Fill each Mason jar to the very top, or until all the vegetables are covered. Secure the lid loosely, and store in a cool, dark place.

4) Each day, open the jar to release the fermenting gases. Cover, shake, and seal the jar again loosely. Do this for 5 days. After the fifth day, you can refrigerate the jars. These vegetables will last for up to 1 month.

Visit www.flatbelly365.com/resources for a tutorial video to learn a quick and easy way to make your own fermented vegetables.

Per Serving: 39 Kcal, Protein 1.5g, Carb 8g, Fat 0g, Sodium 1200mg, Dietary Fiber 2g
Daily Values: Fiber 7.4%, Vitamin C 36%, Vitamin A 23%, Vitamin D 0%, Potassium 5%, Calcium 4%, Iron 4%

Basic Quinoa

Servings: 4 ✦ Serving Size: 1 cup

Vegan, Gluten Free

This is a simple, basic quinoa recipe.

INGREDIENTS:

1 cup quinoa

2 cups water

DIRECTIONS:

1) Put the quinoa in a sieve and rinse it under cold water until the water runs clear.

2) Transfer the quinoa to a medium saucepan and add the water. Bring to a boil, cover, and reduce the heat to low.

3) Simmer until all the water has been absorbed, for 15 to 20 minutes. Fluff with a fork and serve.

Note: Quinoa will keep in the refrigerator for 3 to 5 days.

Per Serving: 156 Kcal, Protein 6g, Carb 27g, Fat 3g, Sodium 7mg, Dietary Fiber 3g,
Daily Values: Fiber 11%, Vitamin C 0%, Vitamin A 0%, Vitamin D 0% Potassium 5% Calcium 2%, Iron 11%

Roasted Vegetables

Servings: 10 ✦ Serving Size: 1 cup

Vegan, Gluten Free

This is a multicolored roasted vegetable recipe that you can add to soups, pastas, salads, and stews.

INGREDIENTS:

1 medium red onion

1 medium bell pepper

1 medium zucchini

1 medium carrot

2 cups Brussels sprouts

1 head cauliflower, florets only

1 tablespoon olive oil

1½ teaspoons sea salt

½ teaspoon black pepper

DIRECTIONS:

1) Preheat the oven to 450° F.

2) Chop all the vegetables into pieces of equivalent size, about 1 to 2 inches.

3) Put the chopped vegetables in a roasting pan with the oil and season with salt and pepper. Toss to combine.

4) Roast the vegetables for 20 minutes, or until they are tender and their edges are browned.

Note: Roasted vegetables will keep in the refrigerator for 3 to 5 days.

Per Serving: 50 Kcal, Protein 2g, Carb 8g, Fat 1.6g, Sodium 291mg, Dietary Fiber 2.5g
Daily Values: Fiber 9%, Vitamin C 83%, Vitamin A 13%, Vitamin D 0%, Potassium 7%, Calcium 2%, Iron 4%

Cannellini (White) Beans

Servings: 4 ✦ Serving Size: 1½ cups

Vegan, Gluten Free

This is a classic recipe for cooking dry beans from scratch. It's not as hard as you think. You can cook most varieties of dried beans using this technique, too.

INGREDIENTS:

1 pound cannellini beans

4 cups stock *(vegetable, chicken, or beef)*

Salt and pepper, to taste

DIRECTIONS:

1) Put the beans in a stockpot and cover them with 3 inches of water. Let them soak for 4 hours. Drain the beans in a colander and discard the water.

2) Transfer the beans back to the stockpot and cover with 3 inches of water again. Bring to a boil over medium heat. Drain the beans in a colander and discard the water. This process helps remove the oxalates in beans, which are responsible for gastrointestinal discomfort.

3) Transfer the beans back to the stockpot and add the stock. Season the beans with salt and pepper, to taste. Cover, lower the heat, and cook the beans at a simmer for about 1 hour or until they are soft. Serve warm.

Note: The beans will keep in the refrigerator for 3 to 5 days and may be reheated as needed.

Per Serving: Kcal 400, Protein 29g, Carb 71g, Fat 1g, Sodium 1897mg, Dietary Fiber 29g,
Daily Values: Fiber 102%, Vitamin C 6%, Vitamin A 0%, Vitamin D 0% Potassium 40% Calcium 14%, Iron 54% 68%

Gut-Healing Overnight Oats

Servings: 6 ✦ Serving Size: ²/₃ cup

Vegetarian

This warm and delicious breakfast on the go is not only quick to piece together, but it's an easy way to start your day. Oats and apples are loaded with soluble fiber, which is essential for gut health, while walnuts are known prebiotics that have been shown to promote beneficial gut bacteria while lowering bad gut bacteria through their significant amount of plant-based omega-3s and fiber.

INGREDIENTS

2 cups oats, dried

2 cups 1% milk

½ cup applesauce, unsweetened

½ cup nonfat Greek yogurt

¼ cup prunes, diced

¼ cup walnuts, chopped

1 tablespoon vanilla extract

1 teaspoon cinnamon powder

¼ teaspoon sea salt

A growing body of evidence suggests that prunes can have a positive impact on bone health. Prunes contain a variety of nutrients that play a role in bone building and structure, like maintenance, vitamin k, phosphorus, boron, and potassium.

DIRECTIONS

1) Put all ingredients in a storage container. Mix together and let sit overnight for at least 6 hours. Stir before each use.

Per Serving: Kcal 312, Protein 15g, Carb 47g, Fat 8g, Sodium 118mg, Dietary Fiber 7g,
Daily Values: Fiber 24%, Vitamin C 0%, Vitamin A 6%, Vitamin D 5%, Potassium 10%, Calcium 12%, Iron 16%

Miso Roasted Tofu

Servings: 6 ✦ Serving Size: 1 slice

Vegan

Prep the tofu on a weekend and use it throughout the week. Add to salads, grain dishes, vegetables dishes, or any dish where you want some extra protein.

INGREDIENTS:

1 tablespoon red miso

2 cloves garlic, crushed

2 tablespoons white vinegar

1 tablespoon Bragg's amino acids *(substitute low sodium soy sauce)*

1 (14 oz) block extra firm tofu, drained

Canola oil spray

DIRECTIONS:

1) Preheat the oven to 400°F.

2) Place the red miso, garlic, vinegar, and Bragg's amino acids in a large, shallow bowl. Mix them with a fork to create a smooth, homogenous mixture. Set aside.

3) Slice drained tofu into six ½-inch slabs. Dip each piece of tofu in the marinade, making sure to coat all sides completely. Let the tofu rest in the marinade for 30 minutes (tofu can also be left to marinate overnight in the refrigerator for convenience).

4) Lightly spray a small roasting pan with oil. Place each piece of tofu in the pan, ½-inch apart. Pour the remaining marinade over each piece of tofu.

5) Bake for 30 minutes or until the tofu is crisp and golden around the edges. Let cool slightly before serving.

6) Roasted tofu can be stored in the refrigerator for 3 to 5 days, and may be eaten hot or cold.

Per Serving: Kcal 73, Protein 7g, Carb 3g, Fat 4g, Sodium 220mg, Dietary Fiber 0g,
Daily Values: Fiber 1%, Vitamin C 0%, Vitamin A 0%, Vitamin D 0% Potassium 2% Calcium 9%, Iron 7%

Oregano Roasted Chicken

Servings: 6 ✦ Serving Size: 4 ounces

Gluten Free

Make this recipe on a Sunday so that you have chicken to use whenever you need it throughout the following week. You can use this chicken in multiple recipes from this book. It can be added to salads, soups, grain dishes, and more.

INGREDIENTS:

1½ pounds skinless chicken breasts

Juice of 1 lemon *(about 3 tablespoons)*

1 tablespoon canola oil

¼ cup dry oregano

1 tablespoon garlic powder

Salt and pepper, to taste

DIRECTIONS:

1) Preheat the oven to 450°F.

2) Place the chicken breasts in a roasting pan. Pour the juice and oil over the breasts and toss them to coat. Sprinkle the chicken breasts with the oregano, garlic powder, and salt and pepper, to taste.

3) Bake the chicken for 22 minutes or until crisp and golden on the outside and moist on the inside. Remove it from the oven and let it cool for 5 to 10 minutes before slicing.

Note: The chicken keeps well in the refrigerator for 3 days.

Per Serving: Kcal 151, Protein 23g, Carb 4g, Fat 5g, Sodium 303mg, Dietary Fiber 2g,
Daily Values: Fiber 6%, Vitamin C 3%, Vitamin A 1%, Vitamin D 0% Potassium 8% Calcium 4%, Iron 9%

Chicken Parsley Burger

Servings: 8 ✦ Serving Size: 1 patty (5 oz/140 g)

Gluten Free

This chicken patty, seasoned with parsley, garlic, and onions, is perfect for summertime. Cooking with canola oil allows the great flavors of the herbs to stay intact, while resisting the high heat of the sauté pan and the grill. Enjoy this chicken patty as a burger, on top of a salad, or paired with rice and bean bowls. Rainy outside? Not a problem. You can use a griddle or frying pan for easy and efficient indoor cooking.

INGREDIENTS:

1 tablespoon canola oil

1 cup red onion, diced

½ cup parsley, finely chopped

2 teaspoons garlic, minced

2 pounds lean ground chicken

1 teaspoon sea salt

¼ teaspoon ground black pepper

Canola oil spray

DIRECTIONS:

1) Heat a sauté pan on medium heat. Place the canola oil in the pan and let it heat up for about 1 minute. Add the onion and parsley and sauté for about 3 minutes or until the onions become translucent. Add the garlic and cook for an additional 1 minute. Remove from the heat and let cool for about 3 minutes.

2) In a large bowl, place the ground chicken, salt, pepper, and parsley mixture. Mix well.

3) With your hands, form eight (5 oz/140 g) patties and set them aside in a baking sheet.

4) Heat the grill to medium high heat (medium if using an indoor griddle or frying pan). Spray the grill with canola oil spray. Place the chicken patties on the grill and cook for 5 minutes on each side or until they are done.

Per Serving: Kcal 190, Protein 20g, Carb 2g, Fat 11g, Sodium 294mg, Dietary Fiber 0g,
Daily Values: Fiber 0%, Vitamin C 8%, Vitamin A 2%, Vitamin D 0% Potassium 14% Calcium 1%, Iron 7%

Thyme-Rubbed Lamb Chops

Servings: 6 ✦ Serving Size: 3 ounces of lamb

Gluten Free

This is a quick and delicious way to cook lamb and provides a satisfying amount of protein and rich flavor.

INGREDIENTS:

6 lamb loin chops, bone-in—3x2 inch pieces, 5 ounces each

1 tablespoon cumin

1 tablespoon coriander

½ teaspoon black pepper

1 teaspoon sea salt

1 teaspoon garlic

2 teaspoons thyme leaves

Supporting a strong immune system begins with a healthy diet. A single portion of lean lamb serves up a significant amount of nutrients essential for immune function: zinc, selenium, protein, and iron.

DIRECTIONS:

1) Mix the cumin, coriander, pepper, salt, garlic, and thyme in a bowl. Add lamb and toss to coat.

2) Place lamb on grill and cook for 4 minutes on each side.

Per Serving: Kcal 150, Protein 23 g, Carb 0 g, Fat 6 g, Sodium 198 mg, Dietary Fiber 0 g,
Daily Values: Fiber 0%, Vitamin C 0%, Vitamin A 0%, Vitamin D 0.8% Potassium 12% Calcium 1%, Iron 20%

Grilled Lemon Salmon

Servings: 4 ✦ Serving Size: 4 oz.

Gluten Free

This recipe is a basic way to grill salmon for any occasion. It can be added to salads and grain bowls. You can use a griddle or frying pan for easy and efficient indoor cooking.

INGREDIENTS:

1 pound salmon with skin

4 cloves garlic, crushed

3 tablespoons lemon juice

1 teaspoon sea salt

½ teaspoon black pepper

DIRECTIONS:

1) Place the salmon, skin side down, in a casserole dish. Cover with the garlic, lemon juice, salt, and pepper. Let the salmon marinate at room temperature for 30 minutes.

2) Meanwhile, heat your grill according to the manufacturer's instructions.

3) Grill the salmon, turning as necessary until the fish turns opaque and flakes when pulled apart with a fork. Serve immediately.

Per Serving: Kcal 113, Protein 20g, Carb 2g, Fat 6g, Sodium 430mg, Dietary Fiber 0g,
Daily Values: Fiber 0%, Vitamin C 5%, Vitamin A 1%, Vitamin D 0% Potassium 11% Calcium 1%, Iron 5%

Lemon-Roasted Fish

Servings: 4 ✦ Serving Size: 1 fillet (5 oz.)

Gluten Free

This is a basic recipe for roasting fish—quick, easy, and simple. The fish can be added to salads and grain bowls.

INGREDIENTS:

4 fillets white fish *(sea bass, tilapia, or sole)*

Juice of 1 lemon *(about 3 tablespoons)*

1 lemon, whole

1 tablespoon olive oil

Salt and pepper, to taste

DIRECTIONS:

1) Preheat the oven to 375°F.

2) Place the fillets in a roasting pan and coat them with the lemon juice, oil, salt, and pepper, to taste.

3) Slice the whole lemon into thin rounds, and remove the seeds from each slice. Distribute the slices equally among the fish fillets.

4) Roast the fillets for 15 to 25 minutes (depending on the thickness of the fillets) until the fish is white and flakes when pulled apart with a fork. Serve immediately.

Per Serving: Kcal 142, Protein 22g, Carb 3g, Fat 5g, Sodium 394mg, Dietary Fiber 1g,
Daily Values: Fiber 4%, Vitamin C 21%, Vitamin A 0%, Vitamin D 17% Potassium 8% Calcium 2%, Iron 5%

Spiced Turmeric Milk

Servings: 1 ✦ Serving Size: ¾ cup

Vegetarian/Gluten Free

This spiced drink is packed with anti-inflammatory and antioxidant properties found in turmeric, ginger, and cinnamon. In India, this "Golden Milk" is made with real cow's milk. For some people, like me, it can be difficult to consume milk due to digestive problems linked to lactose intolerance. Or so I thought. Recently, I discovered a2 Milk® and have used it in many of my recipes, without any digestive discomfort. a2milk® is the only cow's milk in the U.S. market that is free from the A1 beta-casein protein. This protein has been linked to inflammation and digestive discomfort, similar to lactose intolerance. All cows naturally produce either A1 or A2 beta-casein proteins, or a combination of both, in their milk. By using a simple hair follicle test, they're able to determine which protein each cow is producing. If a cow is found to be producing only A2 beta-casein, it is separated from the rest of the herd for its milk (see the color photo page 178).

INGREDIENTS:

1 cup 2% a2 Milk®
½ teaspoon turmeric powder
1 (½-inch) piece ginger, thinly sliced, or ¼ teaspoon ginger powder
1 cinnamon stick
1 tablespoon honey
cinnamon powder, to garnish

DIRECTIONS:

1) Place the milk, turmeric, ginger, cinnamon stick, and honey in a small saucepan over medium heat. Stir all the ingredients and bring to a low boil.

2) Lower the heat to low and simmer, stirring frequently, for 10 minutes.

3) Serve hot and top with the powdered cinnamon.

Per Serving: Kcal 207, Protein 10g, Carb 32g, Fat 5g, Sodium 146mg, Dietary Fiber 0.4g
Daily Values: Fiber 1.3%, Vitamin C 3%, Vitamin A 0%, Vitamin D 12%, Potassium 10%, Calcium 27%, Iron 5%

Citrus Raspberry Chia Seed Pudding

Servings: 4 ✦ Serving Size: ½ cup

Vegan, Gluten Free

Super simple to prepare. The pudding is not extremely sweet and is very nice on the palate. Experience a light dessert to simply satisfy your sweet tooth (see the color photo page 177).

INGREDIENTS:

1 cup low-fat vanilla almond milk

3 tablespoons chia seeds

1 teaspoon orange zest

⅛ teaspoon ground cinnamon

1 cup raspberries

DIRECTIONS:

1) Place almond milk, chia seeds, orange zest, and cinnamon in a small bowl and whisk to combine. Fold in raspberries. Cover and refrigerate for 2 hours or until firm and pudding-like.

2) Pudding will keep in the refrigerator for 2 to 3 days.

Per Serving: Kcal 84, Protein 3g, Carb 12g, Fat 4g, Sodium 38mg, Dietary Fiber 6g,
Daily Values: Fiber 22%, Vitamin C 10%, Vitamin A 4%, Vitamin D 3% Potassium 2% Calcium 13%, Iron 5%

Baked Apples with Cinnamon and Chia

Servings: 4 ✦ Serving Size: ½ apple

This dessert is fast and effortless and perfect to make for a party or to just enjoy as an after-dinner treat. Your entire family will devour this fruity dessert (see the color photo page 176).

INGREDIENTS:

Canola oil spray

2 large apples, halved

1 tablespoon coconut oil, melted

2 tablespoons agave syrup

2 tablespoons rolled oats

1 tablespoon chia seeds

1 teaspoon cinnamon

DIRECTIONS:

1) Preheat oven to 350°F.

2) Lightly coat a small casserole dish with oil spray. Place apple halves into the dish, cut side up. Remove the center of the apple, including core and seeds, using a melon baller. Bake, uncovered, for 15 minutes.

3) In the meantime, combine coconut oil, agave, oats, chia seeds, and cinnamon in a small bowl. When 15 minutes have passed, remove the apples from the oven. Spoon the filling into the center of each apple.

4) Place the apples back in the oven and continue cooking them until they are tender, for about 15 to 20 minutes longer.

5) These apples will keep in the refrigerator for 1 to 2 days.

Per Serving: Kcal 158, Protein 1g, Carb 26g, Fat 6g, Sodium 1mg, Dietary Fiber 4g,
Daily Values: Fiber 14%, Vitamin C 2%, Vitamin A 0%, Vitamin D 0% Potassium 3% Calcium 2%, Iron 3%

CHAPTER 8

Beyond Flat-Belly 365— Long-Term Success and Maintenance

Congratulations! You've made it to the final phase of the Flat-Belly 365 plan, which is to maintain your flat belly and weight loss goals throughout your daily life. This phase emphasizes the positive patterns and habits you need to develop to maintain lifelong success with your health and wellness. By following these guidelines, you'll experience amazing antiaging benefits. You will be full of energy, vitality, and internal strength. Your body will appreciate all the superfoods you consume on a daily basis.

Female Plan

For women, you will increase your overall food intake by 25 percent of your original 1,300-calorie flat belly plan. What this means is that throughout the day, you will be adding additional food to your meals and snacks to maintain the weight you have achieved.

For example:

Add a piece of fruit at breakfast or as a snack (1 more fruit per day).

Add 2 ounces of protein at lunch and dinner (4 oz per day).

Add ¼ cup of extra grain or starch at lunch and dinner (½ cup total per day).

Continue to consume your pre-exercise shake (keep as active as you can to
  help maintain your success).

By adding in these extra food sources, you will increase your intake by 25 percent and maintain your long-term success. Continue to follow the menus and incorporate the other mouthwatering recipes in the book to enjoy a life of variety, diversity, superfoods, and flavor.

Male Plan

For men, you will increase your overall food intake by 35 percent of your original 1,800-calorie flat belly plan. What this means is that throughout the day, you will be adding additional food to your meals and snacks to maintain the weight you have achieved.

For example:

Add ½ cup extra grain and starch at breakfast.

Add a piece of fruit at breakfast and as a snack (2 more fruits per day).

Add 3 ounces of protein at lunch and dinner (6 oz per day).

Add ½ cup of extra grain and starch at lunch and dinner (1 cup total per day).

Continue to consume your pre-exercise shake (keep as active as you can to
  help maintain your success).

By increasing your daily food intake by 35 percent, you can maintain lifelong maintenance and success.

Remember that life is to be enjoyed and no one can be perfect every day. If you feel yourself slipping back into bad habits or if you have over-indulged on vacation or during the holidays, you can do a 7-day reboot at any time.

You have the power to make positive choices every day that will bring you renewed health and vitality. Visit *www.flatbelly365.com/resources* to obtain your downloadable versions of tables, shopping lists, and videos that can enhance your success in achieving and maintaining a lifetime of health.

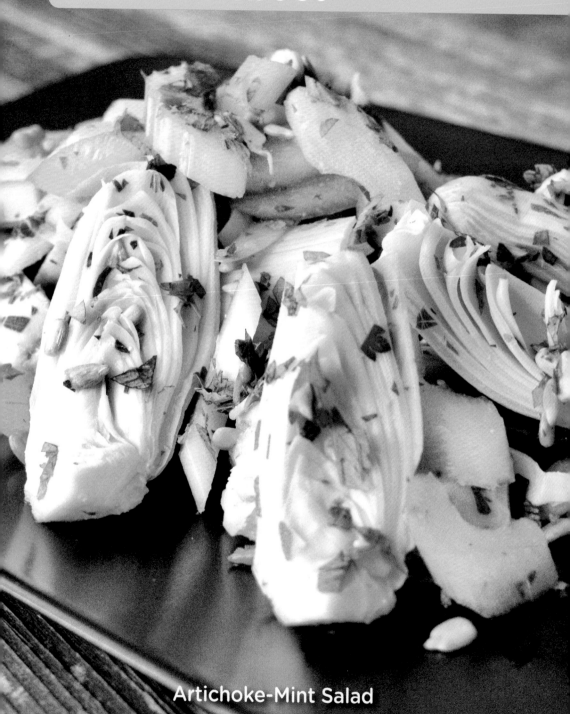

Artichoke-Mint Salad

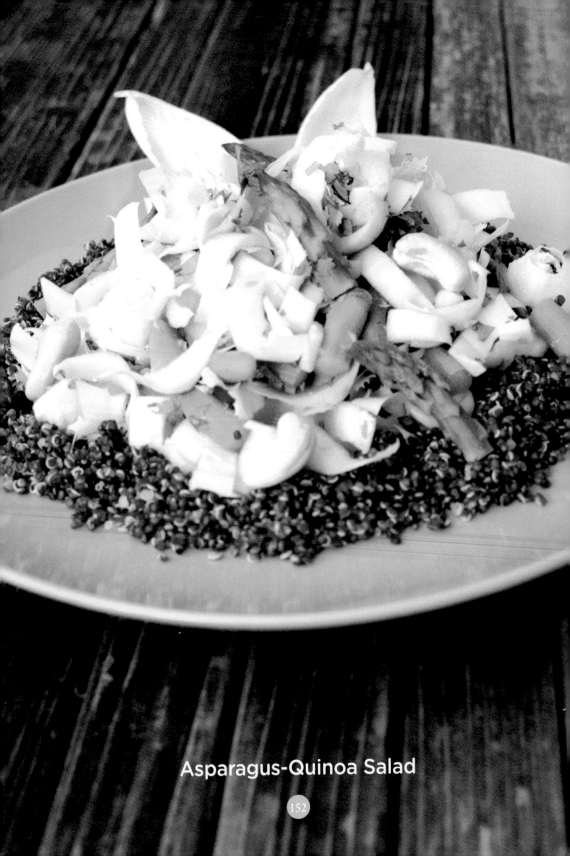

Asparagus-Quinoa Salad

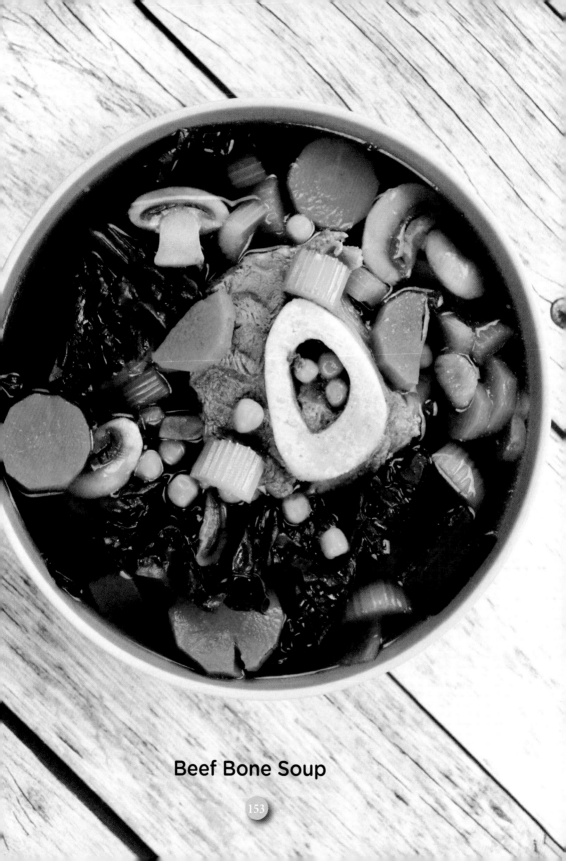

Beef Bone Soup

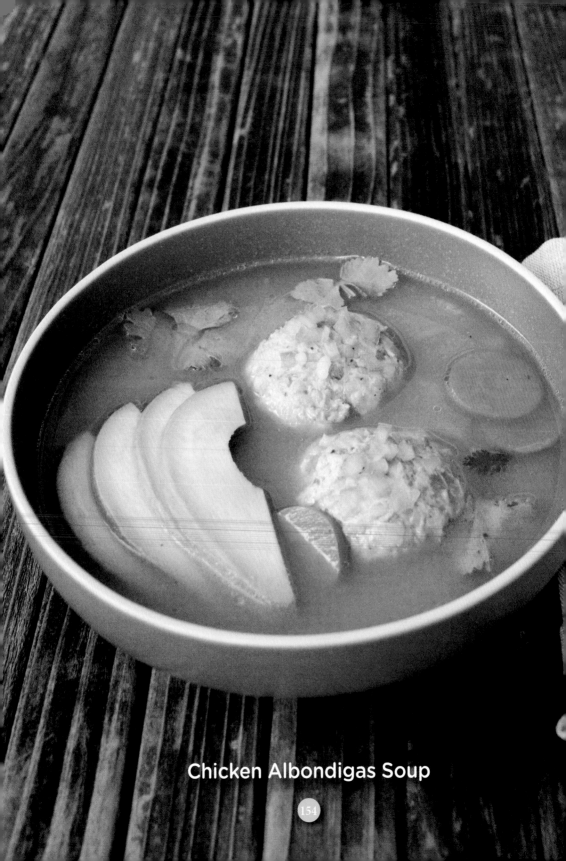

Chicken Albondigas Soup

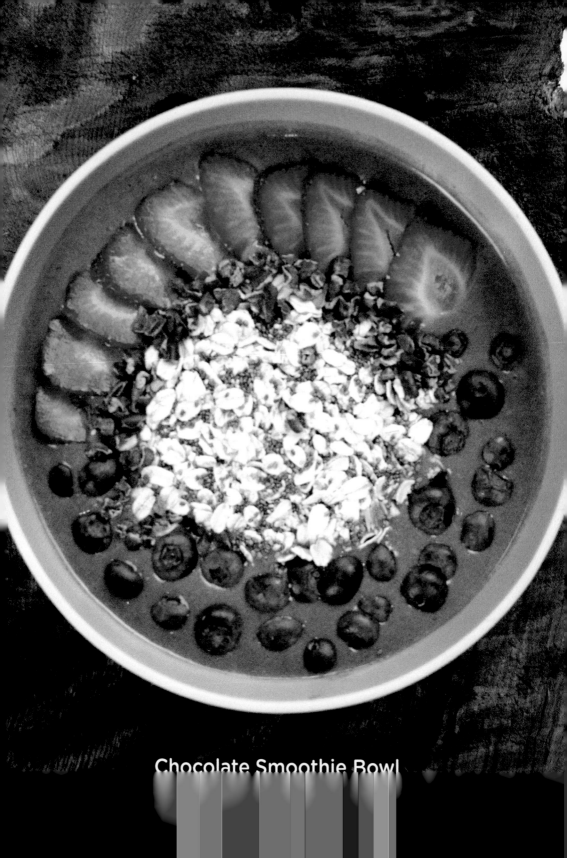

Chocolate Smoothie Bowl

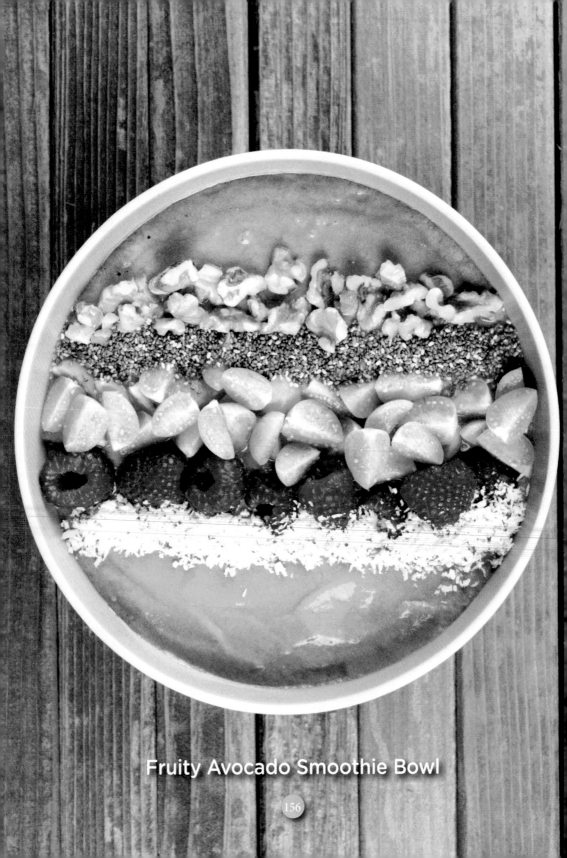

Fruity Avocado Smoothie Bowl

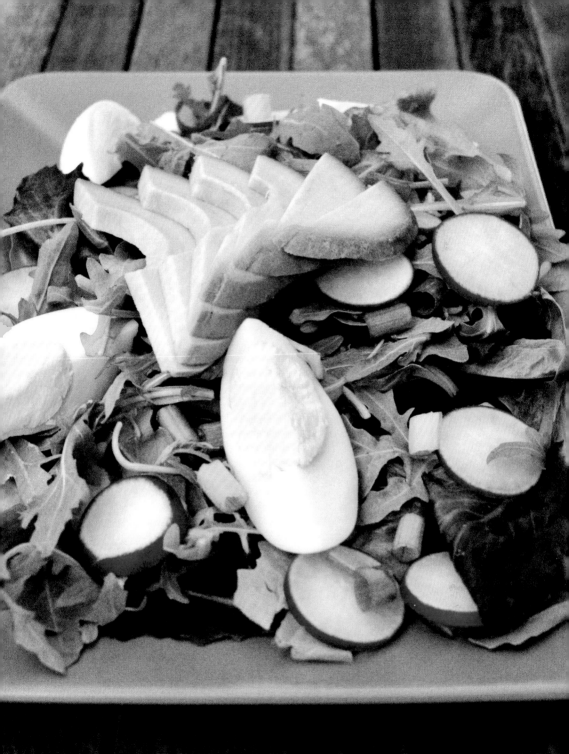

Egg and Avocado Spring Salad

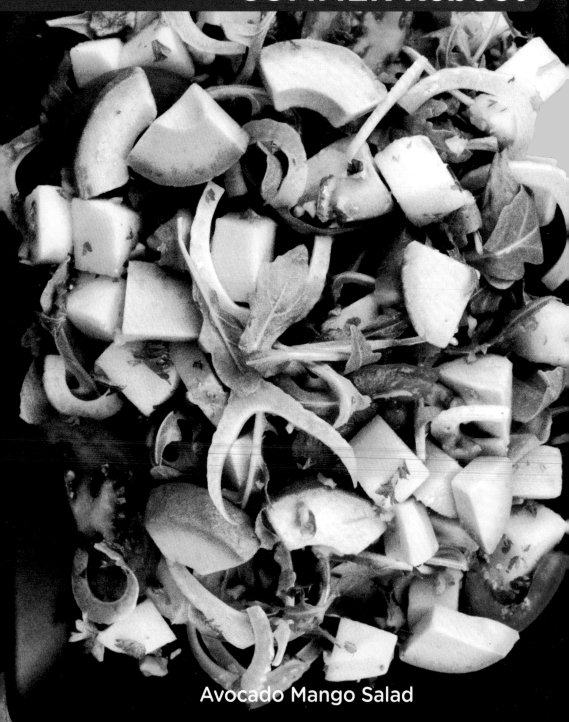

Avocado Mango Salad

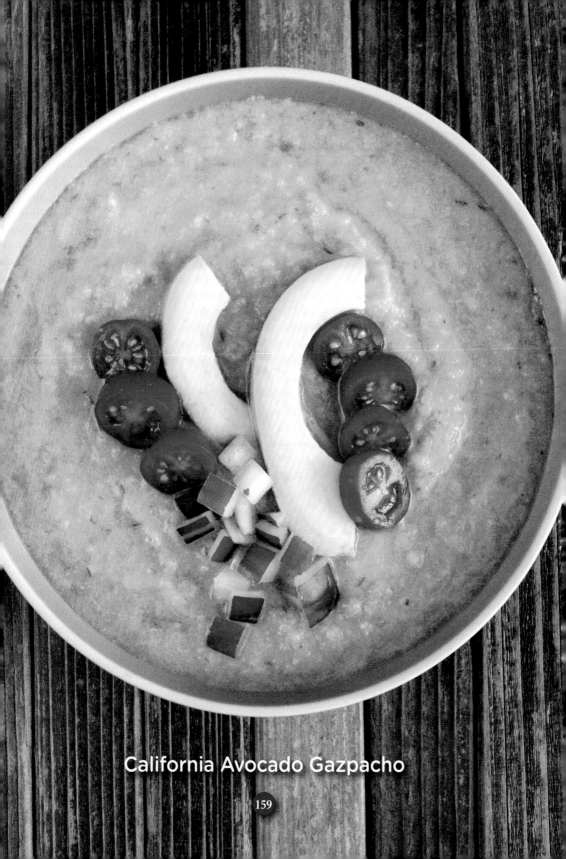

California Avocado Gazpacho

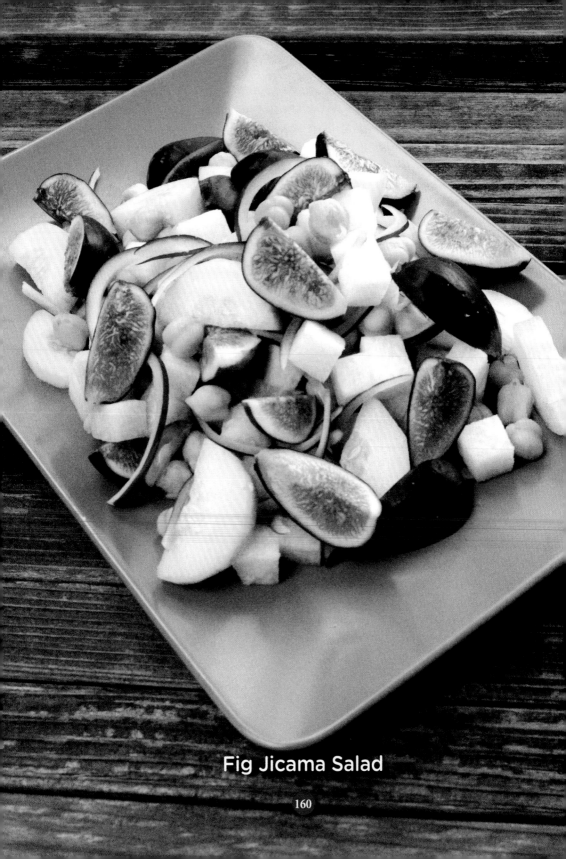

Fig Jicama Salad

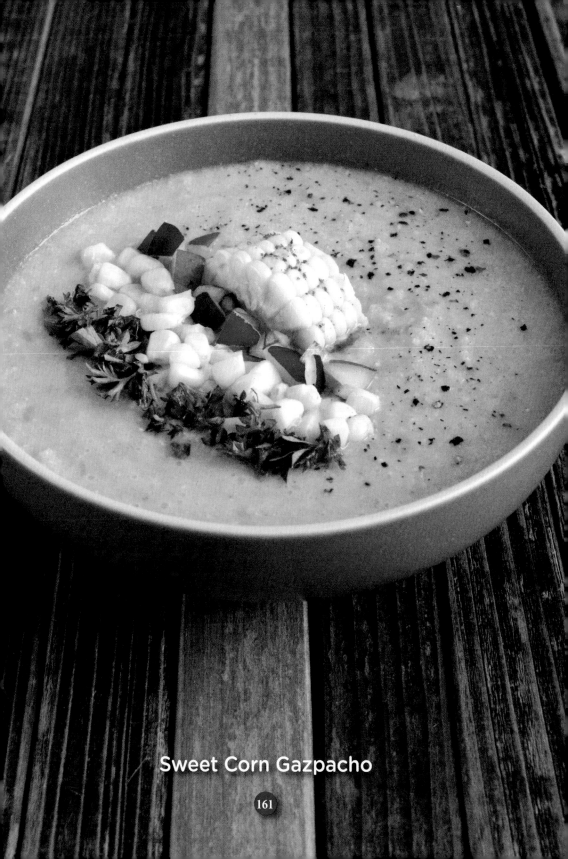

Sweet Corn Gazpacho

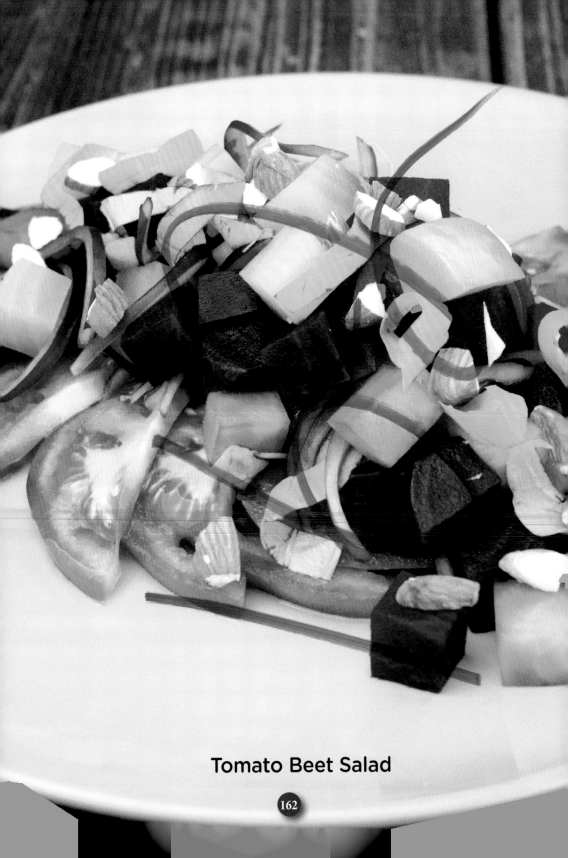

Tomato Beet Salad

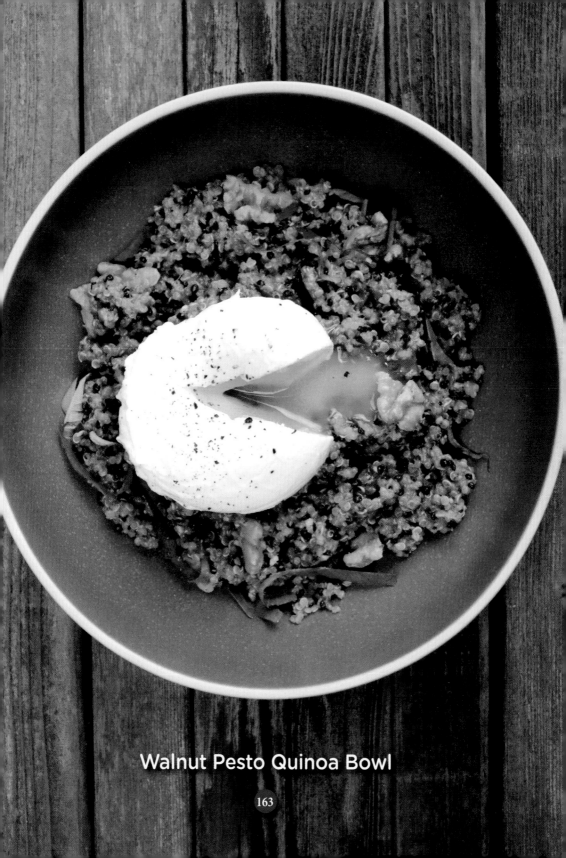

Walnut Pesto Quinoa Bowl

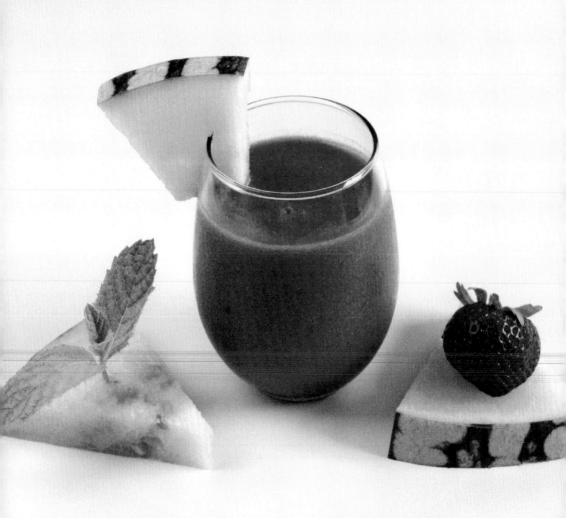

Watermelon Strawberry Smoothie

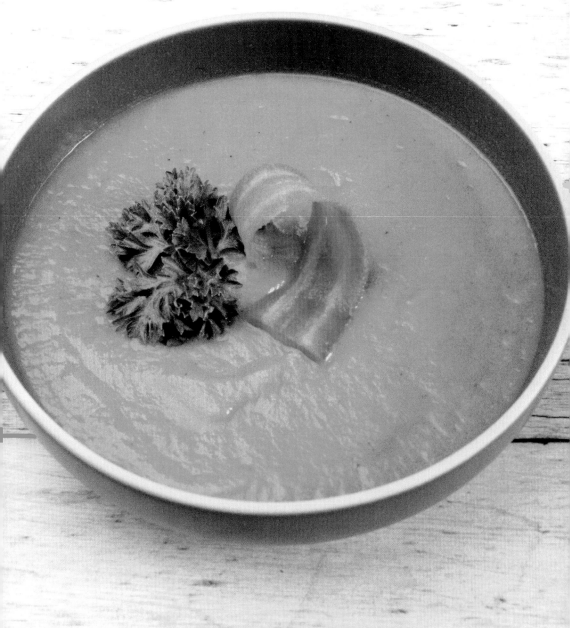

Creamy Butternut Squash Soup

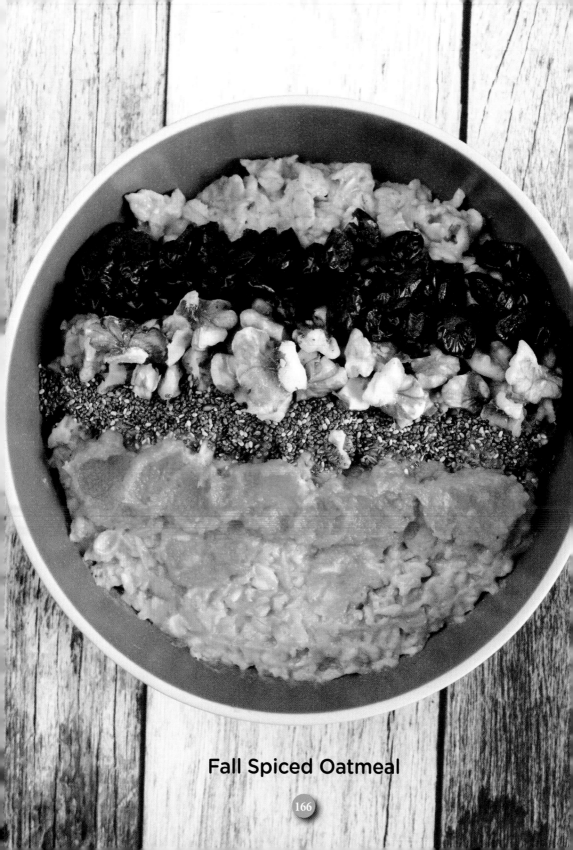

Fall Spiced Oatmeal

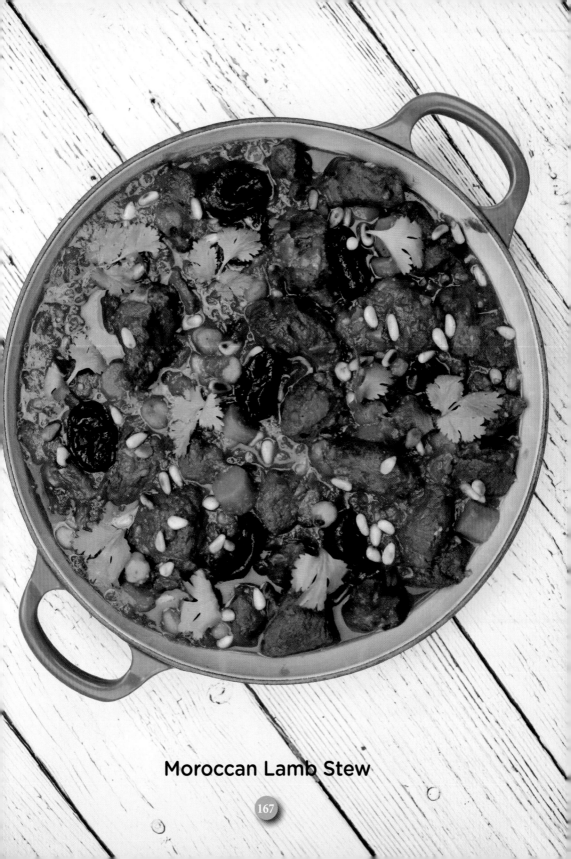

Moroccan Lamb Stew

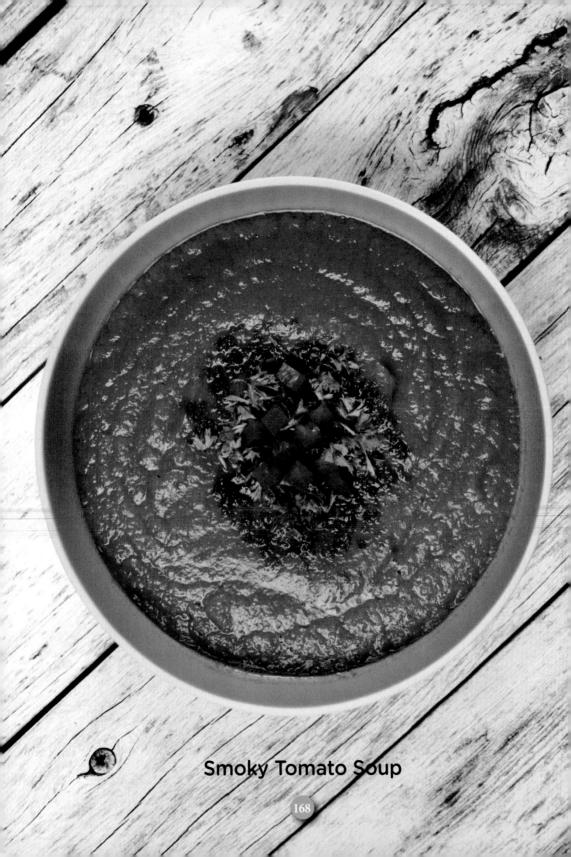

Smoky Tomato Soup

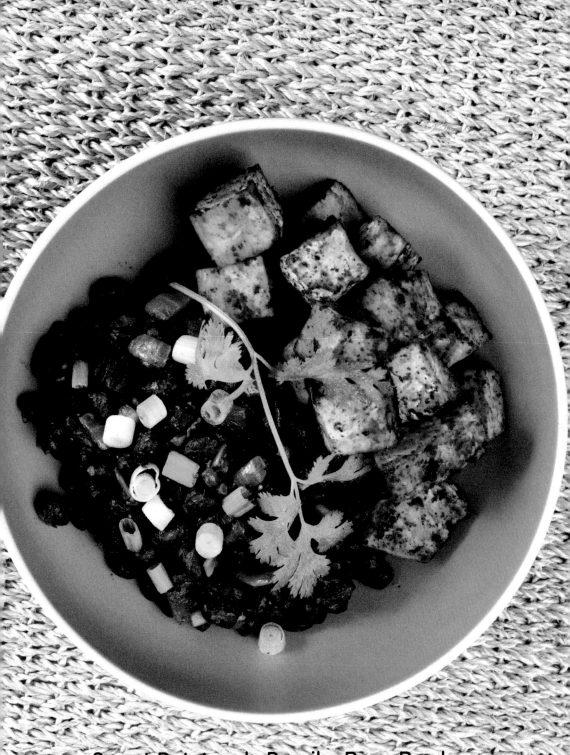

Sweet Potato a la Paprika Bean Bowl

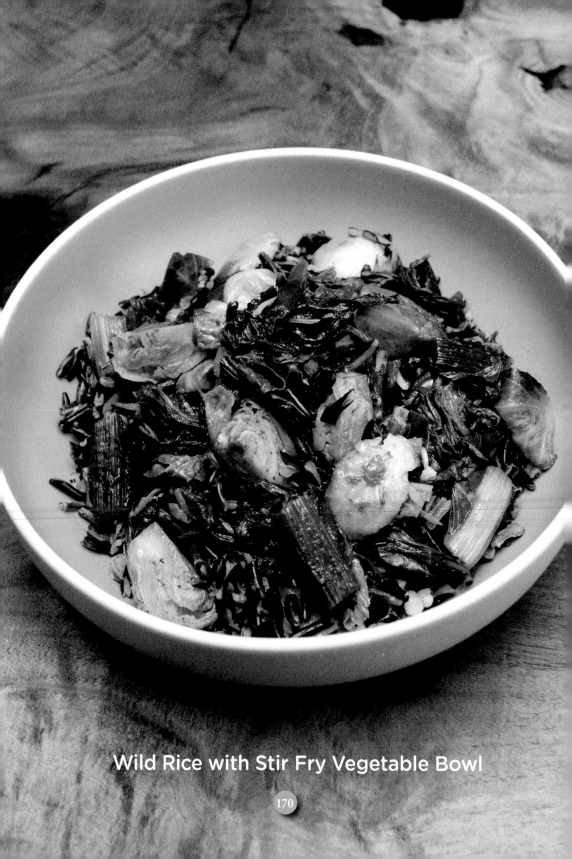

Wild Rice with Stir Fry Vegetable Bowl

Cannellini Chicken Sausage Bowl

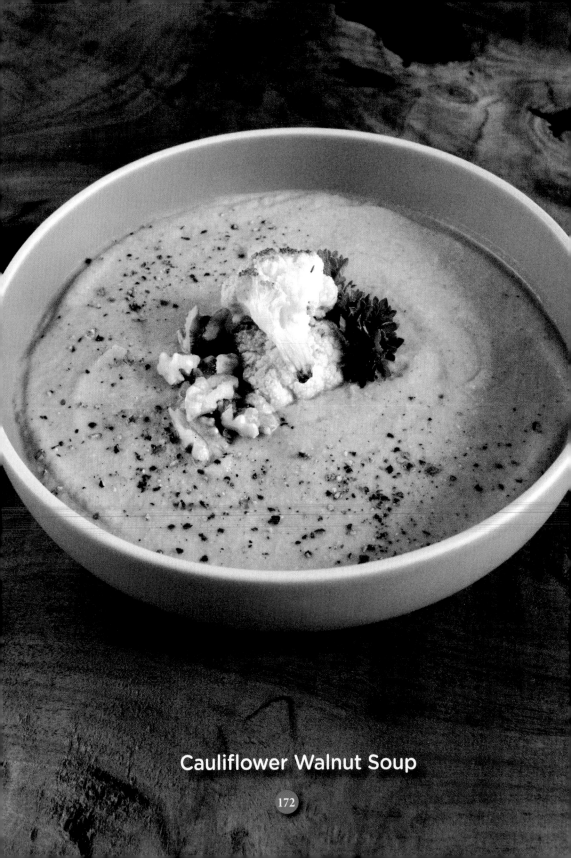

Cauliflower Walnut Soup

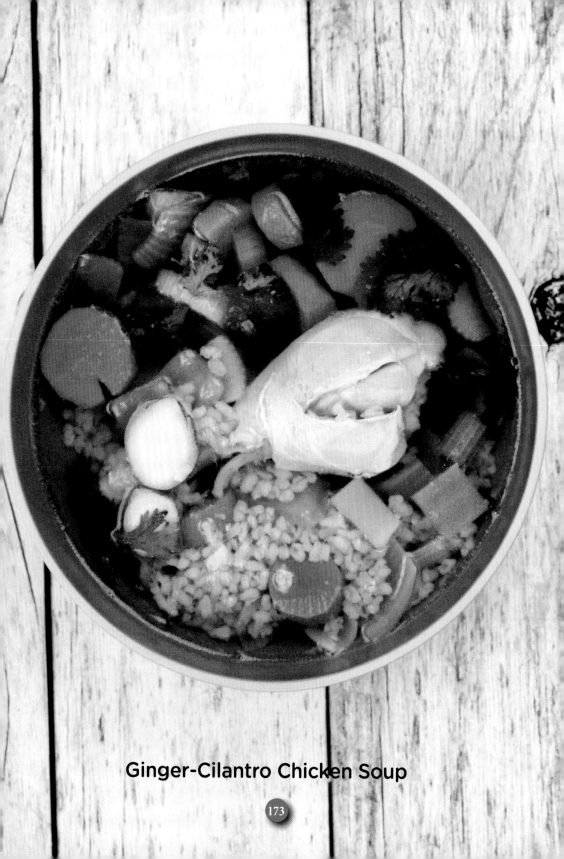

Ginger-Cilantro Chicken Soup

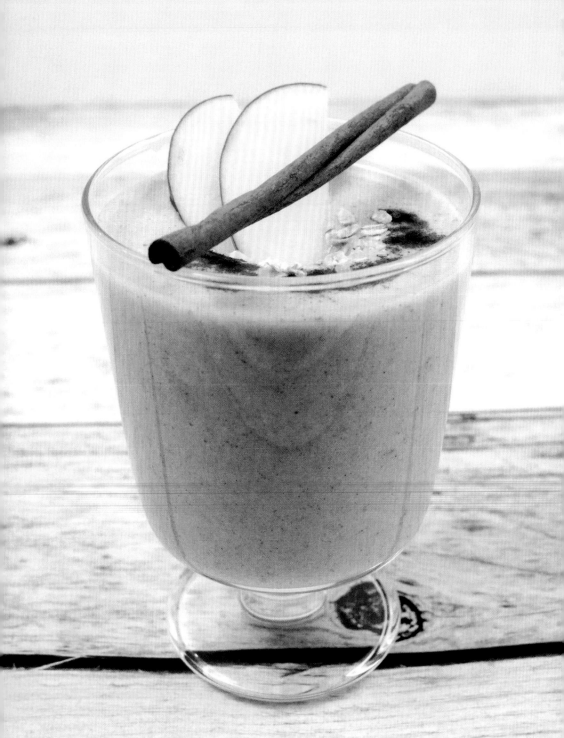

Hot Apple Cinnamon Smoothie

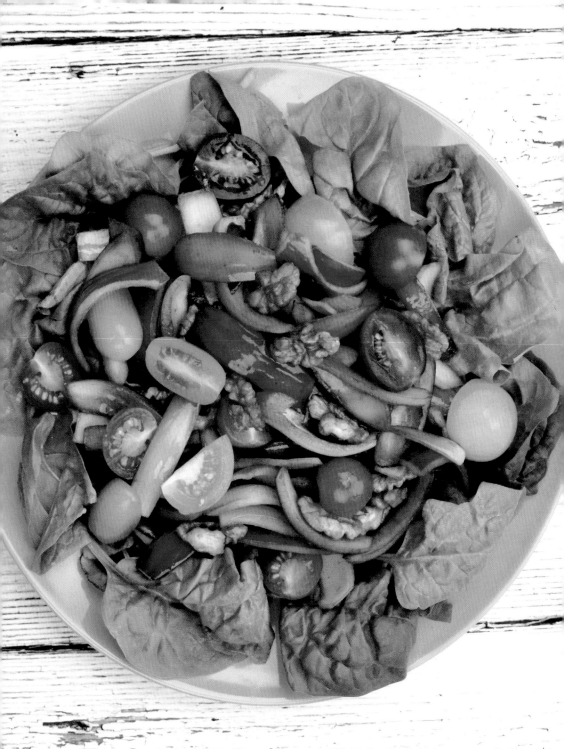

Warm Candied Onion Spinach Salad

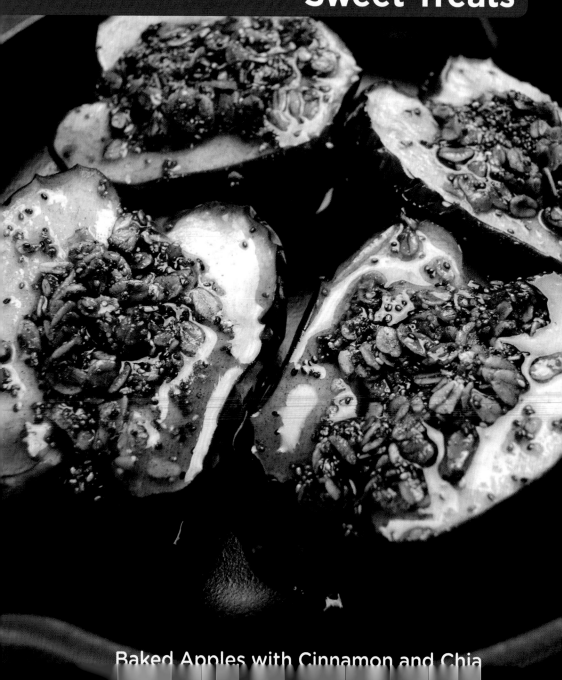

Baked Apples with Cinnamon and Chia

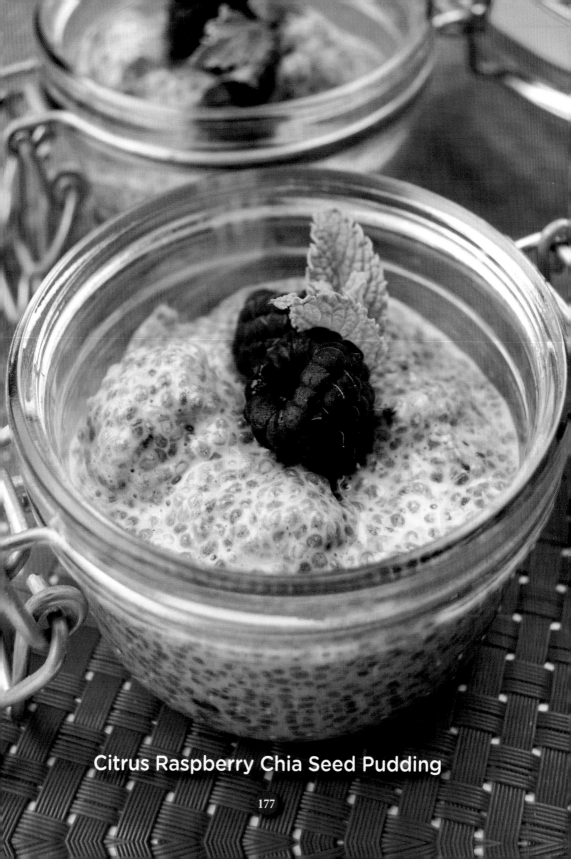

Citrus Raspberry Chia Seed Pudding

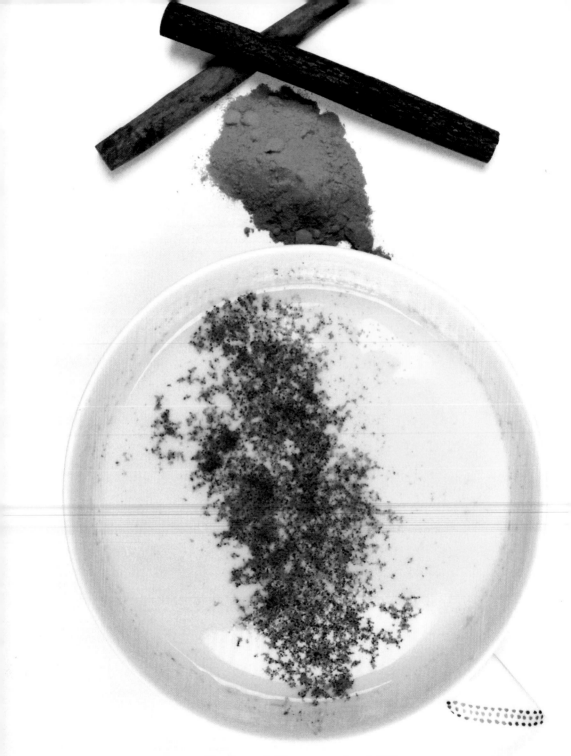

Spiced Turmeric Milk

SOURCES

To access a downloadable version of the references list, *visit www.flat belly365.com/resources*

ABOUT THE AUTHOR

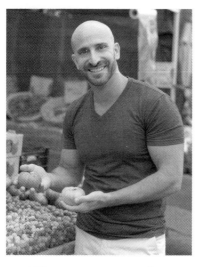

Manuel Villacorta, MS, RDN, is an internationally recognized, award-winning registered dietitian-nutritionist with more than 18 years of experience. He is the author of four books, *Eating Free, Peruvian Power Foods,* and his latest bestseller, *Whole Body Reboot: The Peruvian Superfoods Diet.*

Villacorta is a trusted voice in the health and wellness industry. A national media spokesperson for the Academy of Nutrition and Dietetics from 2010–2013, he is also a health blog contributor for The Huffington Post and an on-air contributor for Univision. Manuel's latest contribution has been as a leading nutrition expert for a series about Superfoods with National Geographic. Additionally, he is a spokesperson for numerous food commodities and companies.

Manuel is the owner of MV Nutrition, a San Francisco-based private practice, and the recipient of five "Best Bay Area Nutritionist" awards from the San Francisco Chronicle, ABC7 News, and Citysearch. Manuel is the founder of the

Whole Body Reboot website & App, a weight loss program with an emphasis on superfoods. He is one of the leading weight loss and nutrition experts in the country.

Born and raised in Peru, he currently lives in San Francisco. Villacorta earned his Bachelor of Science in nutrition and physiology metabolism from the University of California, Berkeley, and his Master of Science in nutrition and food science from California State University, San Jose. He has been the recipient of numerous prestigious awards for his research and contributions to the field of nutrition and dietetics.

INDEX

NOTE: a *t* indicates a table.

A

Alcohol intake tips, 30–31
All season staples, sides, and desserts, 129–145
    Baked Apples with Cinnamon and Chia, 145, 176
    cannellini (white) beans, 134
    Chicken Parsley Burger, 138–139
    Citrus Raspberry Chia Seed Pudding, 144, 177
    fermented vegetables, 130–131
    Grilled Lemon Salmon, 141
    Gut-Healing Overnight Oats, 135
    Lemon-Roasted Fish, 142
    Miso-Roasted Tofu, 136
    Oregano Roasted Chicken, 137
    quinoa, basic, 132
    Spiced Turmeric Milk, 144, 178
    Thyme-Rubbed Lamb Chops, 140
    vegetables, roasted, 133
Anti-oxidant and anti-inflammatory foods, 8–9
Apple Spiced Oatmeal, 116
Artichoke-Mint Salad, 51, 151
Asparagus-Quinoa Salad, 52, 152
Avocado Mango Salad, 76, 158

B

Baked Apples with Cinnamon and Chia, 145, 176
Barley Eggplant Bowl, 120–121
Beef Bone Soup, 57, 153
Belly fat, 6–7
Bowls
    Barley Eggplant Bowl, 120–121
    Cannellini Chicken Sausage Bowl, 118, 171
    Chocolate Smoothie Bowl, 49, 155
    Fruity Avocado Smoothie Bowl, 48, 156
    Sweet Potato a la Paprika Bean Bowl, 96–97, 169
    Walnut Pesto Quinoa Bowl, 80–81, 163
    Wild Rice with Stir Fry Vegetable Bowl, 98–99, 170
Breakfast, 34
Breathing, 36

C

California Avocado Gazpacho, 73, 159
Cannellini Chicken Sausage Bowl, 118, 171
Cannellini (white) beans, 134
Carbohydrates, 10, 12, 18–20
Cauliflower Walnut Soup, 122–123, 172
Chicken
    Cannellini Chicken Sausage Bowl, 118, 171
    Chicken Albondigas Soup, 54–55, 154
    Chicken Parsley Burger, 138–139
    Ginger-Cilantro Chicken Soup, 119, 173
    Oregano Roasted Chicken, 137

Chicken Albondigas Soup, 54–55, 154
Chicken Parsley Burger, 138–139
Chocolate Smoothie Bowl, 49, 155
Chronic inflammation, 7
Cilantro-Lime Dressing, 82
Citrus Raspberry Chia Seed Pudding, 144, 177
Coffee and tea, 29–30
Combine carbohydrates, proteins, and fats, 35
Cooking, 21
Counting food vs. counting calories, 18–20
    grain types, 19
    metabolic hormones, 19
Cravings cheat sheet, 34
Creamy Butternut Squash Soup, 101, 165

D

De-stress, 36
Dining out tips, 38–39

E

Egg and Avocado Spring Salad, 53, 157
80/20 rule, 38
Exercise, 32–34
    high-intensity exercise, 33
    low-intensity exercise, 32
    pre-exercise shake, 33–34

F

Fall reboot, 87–106, 165–170
    Creamy Butternut Squash Soup, 101, 165
    Fall Spiced Oatmeal, 94, 166
    Moroccan Lamb Stew, 102–103
    1,800 calorie 7-day menu, 92–93
    1,300 calorie 7-day menu, 90–91
    Pumpkin Pie Smoothie, 95
    seasonal fruits and vegetables, 88–89t
    shopping list, 104–106
    Smoky Tomato Soup, 100, 168
    Sweet Potato a la Paprika Bean Bowl, 96–97, 169
    Wild Rice with Stir Fry Vegetable Bowl, 98–99, 170
Fall Spiced Oatmeal, 94, 166
Female plan for long-term success and maintenance, 147–148
Fermented foods, 11–12
Fermented vegetables, 130–131
Fiber, 13

Fig Jicama Salad, 75, 160
Fish, salmon
    Grilled Lemon Salmon, 141
    Lemon-Roasted Fish, 142
Flat-belly 365 plan, 15–39
    alcohol intake tips, 30–31
    coffee and tea, 29–30
    counting food vs. counting calories, 18–20
    cravings cheat sheet, 34
    dining out tips, 38–39
    80/20 rule, 38
    high-intensity exercise, 33
    low-intensity exercise, 32
    90/10 rule, 37
    pre-exercise shake, 33–34
    principles, 34–37
    protein options, 23
    protein sources, 24t
    success principles, 20–24
    sweets, 31–32
    topping options, 24, 29t
    vegetarians and vegans, 23
Fruity Avocado Smoothie Bowl, 48, 156

G

Ghrelin levels, 22, 34–35
Ginger-Cilantro Chicken Soup, 120, 173
Grain types, 19
Grilled Fruit and Vegetable Salad, 78–79
Grilled Lemon Salmon, 141
Gut bacteria, 10–11
Gut-friendly superfoods, 5–14
    anti-oxidant and anti-inflammatory foods, 8–9
    belly fat, 6–7
    chronic inflammation, 7
    fermented foods, 11–12
    fiber, 13
    gut bacteria, 10–11
    microbiome, 9–10
    monosaturated fats, 8
    omega-3 fats, 8
    prebiotic and probiotic foods, 14t
    prebiotics, 12–13
    probiotics, 11
    smoking, alcohol, and stress, 13
    subcutaneous fat, 5–6
    visceral fat, 6
Gut-Healing Overnight Oats, 135

H

High-intensity exercise, 33
Hot Apple Cinnamon Smoothie, 114, 174
Hot Chocolate Smoothie, 115
Hydration, 35–36

K

Kefir Hummus, 124

L

Lemon-Mustard Vinaigrette, 56
Lemon-Roasted Fish, 142
Long-term success and maintenance, 147–149
    female, 147–148
    male, 148–149
Low-intensity exercise, 32

M

Male plan for long-term success and maintenance,
    148–149
Metabolic hormones, 19
Microbiome, 9–10
Miso Roasted Tofu, 136
Monosaturated fats, 8
Moroccan Lamb Stew, 102–103

N

90/10 rule, 37

O

Omega-3 fats, 8
1,800 calorie 7-day menu
    fall, 92–93
    spring, 46–47
    summer, 68–69
    winter, 112–113
1,300 calorie 7-day menu
    fall, 90–91
    spring, 44–45
    summer, 66–67
    winter, 110–111
Oregano Roasted Chicken, 137

P

Peach Papaya Smoothie, 71
Portions, 21
Prebiotic and probiotic foods, 14t
Prebiotics, 12–13
Pre-exercise shake, 33–34
Principles, Flat-Belly 365, 34–37
    breakfast, 34
    breathing, 36
    combine carbohydrates, proteins, and fats, 35
    de-stress, 36
    hydration, 35–36
    skipping meals, 35
    sleep, 37
Probiotics, 11
Protein options, 23
Protein sources, 24t
Pumpkin Pie Smoothie, 95

Q

Quinoa, basic, 132

R

Roasted Strawberry Vinaigrette, 83

S

Salads
    Artichoke-Mint Salad, 51, 151
    Asparagus-Quinoa Salad, 52, 152
    Avocado Mango Salad, 76, 158
    Egg and Avocado Spring Salad, 53, 157
    Fig Jicama Salad, 75, 160
    Grilled Fruit and Vegetable Salad, 78–79
    Tomato Beet Salad, 77, 162
    Warm Candied Onion Spinach Salad, 117, 175
Seasonal fruits and vegetables
    fall, 88–89t
    spring, 42–43t
    summer, 64–66t
    winter, 108–109t
Shiitake Bean Sprout Soup, 58
Shopping, 20
Shopping lists
    fall, 104–106
    spring, 64–65
    summer, 84–86
    winter, 125–127

Silky Papaya Smoothie, 50
Skipping meals, 35
Sleep, 37
Smoking, alcohol, and stress, 13
Smoky Tomato Soup, 100, 168
Smoothies
    Chocolate Smoothie Bowl, 49, 155
    Fruity Avocado Smoothie Bowl, 48, 156
    Hot Apple Cinnamon Smoothie, 114, 174
    Hot Chocolate Smoothie, 115
    Peach Papaya Smoothie, 71
    Pumpkin Pie Smoothie, 95
    Silky Papaya Smoothie, 50
    Watermelon Strawberry Smoothie, 70, 164
Snack limitation, 22–23
Soups
    Beef Bone Soup, 57, 153
    Cauliflower Walnut Soup, 122–123, 172
    Chicken Albondigas Soup, 54–55, 154
    Creamy Butternut Squash Soup, 101, 165
    Ginger-Cilantro Chicken Soup, 120, 173
    Shiitake Bean Sprout Soup, 58
    Smoky Tomato Soup, 100, 168
Spiced Turmeric Milk, 144, 178
Spring reboot, 41–62, 151–157
    Artichoke-Mint Salad, 51, 151
    Asparagus-Quinoa Salad, 52, 152
    Beef Bone Soup, 57, 153
    Chicken Albondigas Soup, 54–55, 154
    Chocolate Smoothie Bowl, 49, 155
    Egg and Avocado Spring Salad, 53, 157
    Fruity Avocado Smoothie Bowl, 48, 156
    Lemon-Mustard Vinaigrette, 56
    1,800 calorie 7-day menu, 46–47
    1,300 calorie 7-day menu, 44–45
    seasonal fruits and vegetables, 42–43t
    Shiitake Bean Sprout Soup, 58
    Silky Papaya Smoothie, 50
    spring shopping list, 64–65
Subcutaneous fat, 5–6
Success principles, 20–24
    cooking, 21
    portions, 21
    shopping, 20
    snack limitation, 22–23
    variation, 21
Summer reboot, 63–86, 158–164
    Avocado Mango Salad, 76, 158
    California Avocado Gazpacho, 73, 159
    Cilantro-Lime Dressing, 82

Fig Jicama Salad, 75, 160
Grilled Fruit and Vegetable Salad, 78–79
1,800 calorie 7-day menu, 68–69
1,300 calorie 7-day menu, 66–67
Peach Papaya Smoothie, 71
Roasted Strawberry Vinaigrette, 83
seasonal fruits and vegetables, 64–65t
shopping list, 84–86
Sweet Corn Gazpacho, 74, 161
Tomato Beet Salad, 77, 162
Walnut Pesto Quinoa Bowl, 80–81, 163
Watermelon Strawberry Smoothie, 70, 164
Sweet Corn Gazpacho, 74, 161
Sweet Potato a la Paprika Bean Bowl, 96–97, 169
Sweets, 31–32

T

Thyme-Rubbed Lamb Chops, 140
Tomato Beet Salad, 77, 162
Topping options, 24, 29t

V

Variation, 21
Vegetables, roasted, 133
Vegetarians and vegans, 23
Visceral fat, 6

W

Walnut Pesto Quinoa Bowl, 80–81, 163
Warm Candied Onion Spinach Salad, 117, 175
Watermelon Strawberry Smoothie, 70, 164
Wild Rice with Stir Fry Vegetable Bowl, 98–99, 170
Winter reboot, 107–145, 171–175
    Apple Spiced Oatmeal, 166
    Barley Eggplant Bowl, 120–121
    Cannellini Chicken Sausage Bowl, 118, 171
    Cauliflower Walnut Soup, 122–123, 172
    Ginger-Cilantro Chicken Soup, 120, 173
    Hot Apple Cinnamon Smoothie, 114, 174
    Hot Chocolate Smoothie, 115
    Kefir Hummus, 124
    1,800 calorie 7-day menu, 112–113
    1,300 calorie 7-day menu, 110–111
    seasonal fruits and vegetables, 108–109t
    shopping list, 125–127
    Warm Candied Onion Spinach Salad, 117, 175